Psychology and Sociology Nursing for GNM (1st Year)

Psychology and Sociology Nursing for GNM (1st Year)

Solved Papers with Important Theory (2016–2007)

As per INC Syllabus

Third Edition

Most Authentic and Updated Solved Question Papers

Poonam Sharda
Post Basic BSc Nursing
Baba Farid University of Health Sciences
Faridkot, Punjab, India

JAYPEE
JAYPEE BROTHERS MEDICAL PUBLISHERS
The Health Sciences Publisher
New Delhi | London

JAYPEE **Jaypee Brothers Medical Publishers (P) Ltd**

Headquarters
EMCA House
23/23-B, Ansari Road, Daryaganj
New Delhi 110 002, India
Landline: +91-11-23272143, +91-11-23272703
+91-11-23282021, +91-11-23245672
E-mail: jaypee@jaypeebrothers.com

Corporate Office
4838/24, Ansari Road, Daryaganj
New Delhi 110 002, India
Phone: +91-11-43574357
Fax: +91-11-43574314
E-mail: jaypee@jaypeebrothers.com

Overseas Office
J.P. Medical Ltd
83 Victoria Street, London
SW1H 0HW (UK)
Phone: +44 20 3170 8910
E-mail: info@jpmedpub.com

EU GPSR Authorised Representative
Logos Europe, 9 rue Nicolas Poussin
17000, La Rochelle, France
Phone: +33 (0) 6 67 93 73 78
E-mail: contact@logoseurope.eu

Website: www.jaypeebrothers.com
Website: www.jaypeedigital.com

Psychology and Sociology Nursing for GNM (1st Year)

First Edition: 2013
Second Edition: 2014
Third Edition: **2017**
Reprint: **2026**
ISBN: 978-93-86322-21-0
Printed at: Samrat Offset Pvt. Ltd.

Dedicated to

My Parents

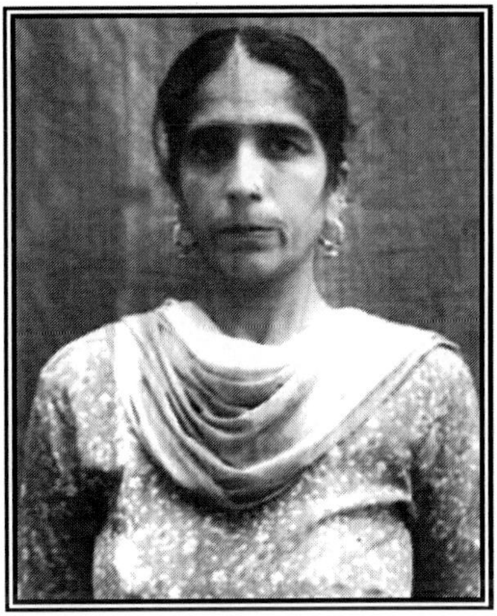

Smt Raj Rani

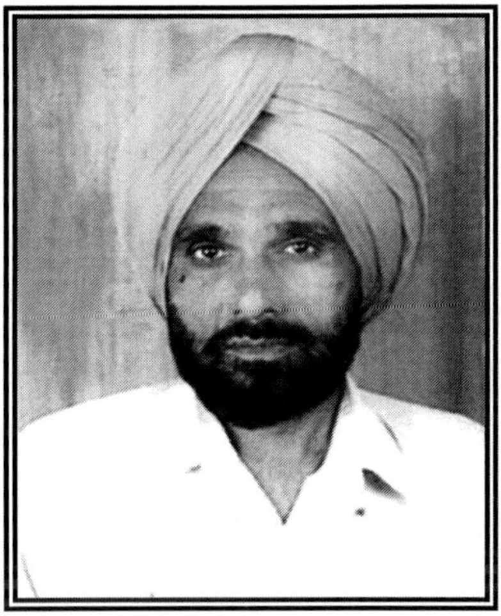

Sh Rajkumar

Preface

It is matter of great pride to present Nursing Solved Question Papers for the first year students of General Nursing and Midwifery (GNM).

As a student, I found difficulty in getting an authentic question bank during my exams. However, there were few books available in the market but they were not having the authentic questions with relevant answers so, I have compiled this question bank which appeared in Baba Farid University of Punjab as per INC regulations.

Psychology and Sociology Nursing for GNM is written with great attention and concentration keeping in mind the basic requirements of Ist year nursing students. It contains solved question papers of Psychology and Sociology Nursing with detailed explanations and important theory given at the beginning of every subject.

I am sure that this book will prove really beneficial to nursing students and will enable them to prepare well for their examination even without books.

Poonam Sharda

Acknowledgments

I am thankful to the God who strengthens me in each and every second in all my work by showing His blessings abundantly through various resources which helped me in accomplishment of the entire task in my life.

My sincere heartfelt thanks to my respected parents Sh Rajkumar and Smt Raj Rani for their help, support and encouragement given to me to achieve this level. Without their help this would not have been possible for me to complete this project.

My sincere thanks goes to Jaypee Brothers Medical Publishers for giving me great opportunity to publish this book.

INC Syllabus

PSYCHOLOGY

Hours: 40

COURSE DESCRIPTION

- This course is designed to help students understand the dynamics of human behavior and concept of mental health. This will enable them to develop positive attitude and good interpersonal relationships in the practice of nursing in all health care settings.

GENERAL OBJECTIVES

Upon completion of this course the students will be able to:

- Describe the concept of mental health and psychology
- Explain the dynamics of human behavior personality and learning
- Discuss the role of adjustment mechanisms and emotions in health and illness
- Demonstrate skills in the application of principle of psychology in nursing practice in all kinds of health care settings.

COURSE CONTENT

Unit I: Introduction

Definitions, scope of psychology and its importance in nursing profession.

Unit II: Psychology of Human Behavior

- Dynamics of behavior, motivation and behavioral process of adjustment, adjustments and maladjustments unconscious behavior
- **Frustration:** Sources and nature of frustration, measures to overcome frustration
- **Conflicts:** Types, unconscious conflict, resolution, conflict and nursing
- **Adjustment mechanism:** Meaning, types and importance
- **Emotions:** In health and disease, emotional situations, control of emotions, effect of emotional reactions on health
- **Attitudes:** Meaning, development, changes in attitude, attitude and nursing

- **Habits:** formation, types, effective habit formation, advantage and disadvantage of habit formation.

Unit III: Learning

- Nature of learning, laws and types of learning, factors promoting
- Effective learning, memory and forgetfulness
- Thinking and type of thinking
- Nature and type of thinking
- Problem-solving and reasoning.

Unit IV: Observation

Attention and perception, factors affection attention and observation and errors in perception.

Unit V: Intelligence

- Definition, individual differences in intelligence
- Mental ability and nature of intelligence
- Measurement of intelligence
- Development of intelligent behavior.

Unit VI: Personality

- **Meaning:** Types, factors affecting development of personality
- **Characteristics of various age group:** Child, adolescent, adult and aged
- Will and character.

SOCIOLOGY

Hours: 20

COURSE DESCRIPTION

This course is designed to help student gain an understanding of sociology in the context of its relevance to nursing practice.

General Objectives

Upon completion of this course, the students will be able to:

- Describe the concept of the family as a social unit and the status of the individual in the family
- Explain the dynamics of society and identify common social problems
- Demonstrate ability to understand the sociocultural and economic aspects of the community in the light of their effects on health and illness

- Utilise the knowledge and understanding of sociology in nursing practice.

COURSE CONTENT

Unit I: Introduction

Concept scope nature and importance of sociology in nursing. The socio-cultural and economic aspects of the community and their effects in health and illness.

Unit II: The Individual

- Brief review of human growth and development
- Effect of environment on childhood, adolescence, adulthood and old age
- The right and responsibilities of the individual in a democratic society.

Unit III: The Family

- Family as a social institution and basic unit for health services
- Basic needs of family, its structure and relationships
- **Family life education:** Pre-marriage, marriage and parenthood.

Unit IV: The Society

- Concept
- **Group:** Types, structure, inter-group relationship. Group cycle, group behavior and group morale
- Social changes, social control, social stratification
- Rural and urban society
- **Social problems:** Unmarried mothers, dowry system, prostitution, drug addiction, alcoholism, delinquency, handicapped, child abuse, women abuse
- Social agencies and remedial measures.

Unit V: The Community

Definition, characteristics and culture.

Unit VI: Economy

- **Resources of the country:** Natural, occupational agricultural, industrial, etc

- Social security
- **Population explosion:** Its effect on economy and the need for population control
- Budgeting for a family, per capital income and its impact on health and illness.

Contents

Important Theory

PSYCHOLOGY

1. Define motivation and types of motives.

Ans. Motivation word is derived from a latin word "movers" which means to propel or to move. Motivation is that internal force that pushes an individual to move toward a goal.

CLASSIFICATION OR TYPES OF MOTIVES

There are three kinds of motives:

1. Primary motive
2. Stimulus motive
3. Secondary or learned motive

These are further divided into:

- **Hunger drive:** When the food supply of the body is exhausted, certain biochemical changes take place in the tissue of the body. The hunger must be satisfied in order to help the body to return to a physiological balance or homeostasis.
- **Thirst drive:** The tissue of the body lose fluid when fluids have not been taken in. As a result, the mucous membranes of the throat become dry and cause sensation of thirst.
- **Respiration drive:** It is drive for air and oxygen. If oxygen is not supplied even for a short time, it is possible to experience brain damage, loss of memory, and control over one's body functions.

Motives

Primary	Stimulus	Secondary
-Hunger driver	Activity	Achievement
-Thirst driver	Curiosity	Affiliation
-Avoidance of pain	Exploration	Aggression
-Need for sleep and air	Manipulation	Power
-Elimination of waste	Physical contact	Curiosity
-Regulation of temperature		
-Sex drive		

- **Sleep drive:** Usually occurs at regular intervals for each person. When the body continues activities without rest or sleep for a long time, it is possible to experience confusion, inability to pay attention, straining, muscle tremors and increased sensitivity.
- **Drive for elimination of wastes:** When the bladder and intestine become distended with waste material, they cause pressure and discomfort. The person becomes restless until the waste materials are disposed.
- **Sex drive:** Unlike hunger, thirst, sex is not essential for the survival of the individual. But it is necessary for the survival of the species.
- **Maternal drive:** Physiological drive causes maternal behavior, maternal drive is caused by prolactin, a hormone secreted by the pituitary.

SOCIAL/SECONDARY MOTIVE

Human beings are not only biological but also social. Therefore, human behavior is activated by the following social motives:

- Achievement
- Affiliation
- Aggression
- Power
- Curiosity.

They are called social motives because they develop through relationship with people.

2. Explain emotions in nursing.

Ans. Nursing is a profession which requires different type of behavioral skills. As a nurse, you should be concerned with the expression and control of emotions.

- In yourself
- In others.

IN YOURSELF

As a nurse, you are the central figure in healthcare. Emotion helps a nurse:

- In understanding oneself, one's conflicts and physical and emotional limits.
- Learn as much as you can, about the causes and physical reactions to emotions. The more you know, better control over emotions you achieve.
- Control stress in your life. Plan your work to avoid emergencies.
- Balance your work with play, exercise and social activities.
- Practice relaxation by meditation, listening to music, reading, dancing or sports.

- Try to control excessive external emotions.
- Use your sense of humor.

CONTROL OF EMOTION IN THE PATIENTS

- **Help the patient to feel welcome:** Give a warm welcome to the patient, let him feel that he is an important guest. Your top priority at the starting of a patient's relationship is to provide a pleasant, relaxed atmosphere.
- **Understand his negative emotions:** Normally, the patients are less self-controlled then the nurses. They are tensed, irritable and unbalanced. The nurse has to be very patience, mature and balanced in her bahavior toward the patient.
- **Promote positive feelings:** She try to eliminate fear, anger, worry, anxiety from patient and develop positive feelings.
- **Develop empathy:** It will be helpful, if the nurse develops empathy with the patient, empathy means understanding the patients situation, feelings and motives. It helps to accept the patient as an individual.
- **Psychosomatic illness:** Patients with a psychosomatic illness may need more of the nurse's time, patience and attention. Such patient needs help to relax and the nurse must arrange professional counseling for such patients when required.

3. Define attention and types of attention.

Ans. The first stage of perception is attention. Attention is the focusing of consciousness on a particular object or idea at the particular time, to the exclusion of other objects or ideas.

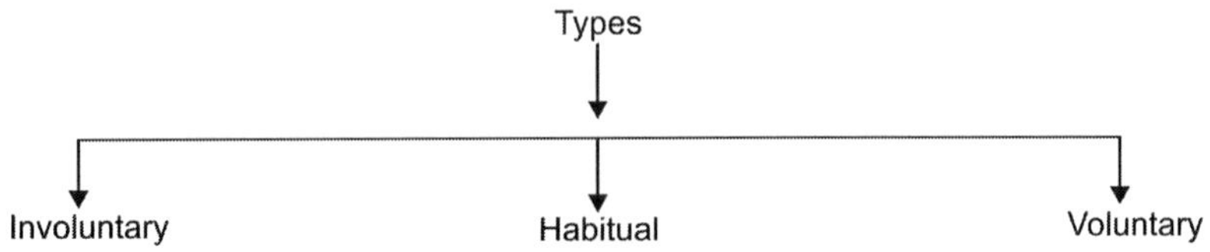

- **Involuntary attention:** It does not require a conscious effort to attend to an object, we give involuntary attention to loud sounds, bright lights, and strong penetration odors.
- **Voluntary attention:** We have to make effort, e.g. uninteresting lectures, difficult assignments.
- **Habitual attention:** There is no conscious effort or sensation, so striking to attract our involuntary attention. We attend to them because of our attitudes, habits or interests, e.g. the attention that a nurse gives to her patients or books on nursing arts.

SPAN OF ATTENTION

The maximum amount of material that can be attended to in one period of attention is called span of attention. If you are able to note all five digits or five letters in a single act of attention, your span of attention is five.

Destruction of Attention

- It refers to shifting of attention from one stimulus to another.

Division of Attention

- It refers to the process of dividing our attention equally between two or more object, e.g. listening to a lecture and writing notes.

4. Describe the factors influencing perception.

Ans.
- Functioning of the sense organs
- Functioning of brain
- Previous experience
- Pregnancy of exposure
- Psychological state of the individual
- Interest
- Motivation
- Behavior of the organism.

5. Explain the types of intelligence.

Ans. Intelligence can be divided into three kinds:
- Mechanical intelligence
- Social intelligence
- Abstract (or general) intelligence.

MECHANICAL INTELLIGENCE

It is the skill to manipulate tools and gadgets in managing the working of machines. Mechanical engineers and trained industrial workers have an abundance of mechanical intelligence.

SOCIAL INTELLIGENCE

It means understanding of people and ability to act wisely in human relationship. Salesmen, diplomats and politicians are supposed to be socially intelligent.

ABSTRACT INTELLIGENCE

It is the ability to handle words, numbers, formulae and scientific principles. A person with abstract intelligence is able to discover relations among symbols to solve problems, e.g. professionals like doctors, lawyers and literary men.

6. Intelligence in relation to sickness.

Ans.
- Intelligence and sickness are related to each other. As intelligence level decreases below average level, it is itself a king of unhealthiness or sickness. Mentally retarded and deficient people are always serious concern for the society.
- Normally, sickness does not directly effect intelligence but because of anxiety or fear, some decline in performance can be observed. It has been observed that strong emotional conditions during sickness can result into blocking of reasoning and rational thinking.
- In case of Down's syndrome and Parkinson's disease, decline in intelligences is observed as important symptom.
- Other disorders like schizophrenia, delusion, hallucinations, also disorganization in cognitive process and it leads strong decline in intelligence.
- In some cases, intelligence helps to facilitate the abnormality of patients, e.g. psychopathic personality is a personality disorder but patient's cognitive functioning remains intact.
- Any decline in intelligence results into various problems and patient finds difficulty in adjusting with sickness. Patient becomes non-cooperative and trouble creator for others. This leads to delay in the recovery of patient, and it creates problem of adjustment in other conditions.

7. Memory in nursing.

Ans. Duty performance of nurse is heavily dependent on memory. She has to remember so many things and matter for better performance. To give better performance and duty efficiently, she has to remember following things:

- Hours of her duty
- Bed numbers in wards
- Name of patient
- Time of medication
- Case history of every patient
- Technical terminology
- Label or brand names of medicine, of few things are taken care according to the nature of working of memory, it can become convenient, it avoids any negligence because of forgetting.

Nurse can also do the following for better performance:

- It is better to keep a diary where important duty matters can be noted.
- It is better to collect elaborated information for any new disease, treatment and medicine.
- Matter too short in length can be forgotten easily, such short length information should be given a little bit special case.
- Various duty matters should be arranged in preference order, based on the significance and seriousness of the matter.
- Various terms and names used in this line are not used in daily life. So, it is better to remember these with attaching meaning. Meaningful terms are remembered better than meaningless.
- Such small tips may help to perform duty more efficiently.

8. Laws of learning.

Ans. There are three laws of learning:

- Law of exercise
- Law of readiness
- Law of effect.

LAW OF EXERCISE

It means if a task is repeated many times, it will be learnt, e.g. if a list of word is read again and again, it will be learnt. The repetition of a task makes the memory strong with practice.

LAW OF READINESS

If an individual is mentally ready to do some task, it will be learnt, e.g. during examination day, the answers of questions are learnt in very short time. So mental readiness helps to learn at better speed and with superior quality.

LAW OF EFFECT

As per law, if some response is rewarded with some prize or benefit, it will be learnt, e.g. if a child is given chocolate for helping others, the child will do that helping behavior again and again. It will be learnt. On other hand, if some behavior is punished, it will be unlearnt, like to punish the child for stealing, the child will stop that bad habit.

9. Change in attitudes.

Ans. Attitudes once developed are difficult to be changed after solidification in adulthood. There are various agencies like government or commercial agencies which political parties use in different ways to change the attitude serving to their interests. Thus, it is always a question as what are the chances of change in attitudes and what factors can make it possible.

CREDIBILITY

Credibility of the source person who is delivering message to change the attitude is very important when the message is delivered by a person who seems to know what they are talking about and to have all the facts do carry more weight than other persons. It increases the credibility of the source and the chances of change in attitude are high.

ATTRACTIVENESS

It is also observed that attractiveness can have strong impact on the attitude of other people and has the power to change it. That's why advertisements are used to deliver the messages.

POWER

A person who is in position and has power can influence others to change their opinion.

DESIGNED MESSAGES

If a message is well-designed according to interest of people, it will help in changing of attitude.

ATTENTION

People are sometime more disposed to get influence for change in attitude when they are distracted by some extraneous events than when they are paying full attention to what is being said to them.

LOW SELF-ESTEEM

People who are low at self-esteem can easily be persuaded for change in attitude than those high on self-esteem. Low esteem person may fell and drown and might not pay attention to messages delivered to them for changing the attitude.

SPEED OF SPEAKING

People who speak rapidly are often more persuasive in changing the attitude.

EMOTIONS

Messages that arouse strong emotions particularly fear are found very effective in changing the attitude.

10. Rules for habit formation.

Ans. William James, the founder of modern psychology in America has given the following rules for habit formation:

- Make a strong start. It helps to have a strong need to develop a habit. A new habit will be formed more quickly if you are very strongly motivated.
- Practice the new habit without exception, until it has been firmly, developed and established in your routines. If you postpone practicing the habit and also allow interruptions in practice, it will be very difficult to establish a new habit.
- Put yourself into situations which will help you develop a habit. Avoid situations that will not help. For example, if you are a late sleeper but want to develop the habit of rising early, you should try to relate with early risers and avoid late sleepers.
- Practice a new habit until it becomes routine then enjoy your new good habit.
- Habits build-up human personality, man should not become a slave to his habits, he should remain the master.

11. Define the following:

- Psychology
- Adjustment
- Motivation
- Frustration
- Conflicts
- Defense mechanism
- Emotions
- Attitudes
- Habit
- Skill
- Learning
- Memory

- Forgetting
- Thinking
- Reasoning
- Attention
- Sensation
- Perception
- Intelligence
- Personality.

PSYCHOLOGY

It is derived from two Greek words "psyche" and "logos" "Psyche" means soul or spirit "logos" means knowledge or study. This is the study of soul. Study of soul or mind is unsatisfactory.

So psychology is defined as the scientific study of behavior and mental processes.

ADJUSTMENT

Adjustment is defined as the continuous process of satisfying one's desires and it involves many aspects of behavior.

MOTIVATION

Motivation derived from a latin word "movere" which means to move motivation is that internal force that pushes an individual to move toward a goal.

FRUSTRATION

When the motives are blocked, frustration occurs, people who cannot achieve their important goals, feel depressed, anxious, fearful, guilty or angry.

CONFLICTS

Conflicts is a special type of frustration. When a person is not able to decide and is confused into two motives is called conflict.

DEFENSE MECHANISM

- ACE investigates to fraud "defense mechanism to refer to the unconscious process that defends (project) a person against anxiety".
- Defense mechanism helps a person to resolve the conflict and reduce the "stress and anxiety" associated with it.

EMOTIONS

It is derived from latin word "emovere which means "stirred up". It is a conscious stirred up state of the organism.

ATTITUDES

It can be defined as mental predisposition of a person to react in a particular manner to others.

HABIT

Habit can be described as an automatic behavior formed by regular repetition of an activity in more or less the some circumstance. Habits can be either good or bad.

SKILL

A skill is a proficiency in performance of a task.

LEARNING

Learning has been defined as a permanent change in behavior that occurs as result of practice or experience.

MEMORY

It can be defined as recalling the material in present learnt in past. For example, student learns a question and then reproduces in exams.

FORGETTING

It is the failure to recall the material learnt in past, e.g. a poem is learnt in morning but when it is recalled in the evening, it is failed.

THINKING

Thinking is a cognitive activity in which verbal, symbols, internal, visual and auditory images, ideas, concepts and mathematical symbols are involved.

REASONING

Reasoning or problem-solving is one of the best forms of controlled thinking in which the thought process is directed consciously toward the solutions of a problem, all facts are arranged in a logical order.

ATTENTION

The first stage of perception is attention; attention is the focusing of consciousness on a particular object or idea at a particular time, to the exclusion of other objects or ideas.

SENSATION

Sensation is the result of physical stimuli operating on our nervous system. The process of sensing, attending and interpreting is called perception.

PERCEPTION

Perception is the interpretation of sensory stimuli which reaches the sense organs and brain.

INTELLIGENCE

Intelligence of a person is his ability to adjust to the world.

PERSONALITY

- The personality is derived from greek word "persona" which means the mask used by factors in greek drama.
- Personality is total quality of an individual's bahavior which is seen in his habits of thinking, in his attitude, interests, his manner of acting and his personal philosophy of life.

SOCIOLOGY

1. Uses of sociology.

Ans.
- Sociology studies lead society in a Scientific way scientific knowledge about human society is needed for progress in various fields of human behaviors.
- Sociology improves our understanding of society, social groups, social institution and their functioning and changing trends help us lead an effective and meaningful social life.
- Sociology helps us to become broad-minded by overcoming our misconceptions, egoism, class, etc.
- Sociology helps us to understand social problems by studying their causes and solutions.
- Social planning has been made easier by sociological study.

- Sociology will improve international understanding.
- Sociology is useful as a teaching subject.
- Sociology has changed our outlook on crime and punishment.

2. Family as a unit of community health service.

Ans. Family as a social institution is the basic unit of health services. It is the focal point of healthcare and the right place for integration, preventive, premotive and curative services. The family system is a basic unit within which the health behavior including health valves, health habits, and health risk perceptions are developed, organized and performed.

The interrelationship between health, health behavior and the family is a highly dynamic one in which each may have a dramatic effect on others.

3. Sex education and its aims.

Ans. Sex education in schools and colleges is necessary to prepare adolescent boys and girls to face the realities of life.

AIMS

- To have the correct knowledge about sex and sexuality.
- To understand and be comfortable with one's own sexuality so as to be able to handle adolescent changes both physical and emotional.
- To establish social relationship with individuals of the same as well as the opposite sex with mutual respect and concern.
- As the first step toward a happy and healthy.

4. Factors affecting social changes.

Ans.
- **Geographical factor:** Changes in the geographical environment create changes in social life. Floods, earthquakes, drought, volcano, eruptions, etc. bring about important changes to society, continuous floods may give rise to new townships.
- **Biological factor:** Intercaste marriages and interrelation marriages produce a new type of human growth with different mental and physical outlook demographic means size and composition of population. A small society may not have a place in history but a large society leaves historical evidence of its culture.
- **Technological factor:** Scientific discoveries inventions and new machineries bring about revolutionary changes in society. For example, the introduction of stream, electric and petrol-driven machines for production-transport and communication has

drastically changed our material environment influencing social changes.

- **Economic factor:** Man has to struggle for his living. There are basic norms that govern the economic relations among people. The mode of production determines the general character of social, political and economic aspects of life.
- **Culture factor:** There is an intimate relationship between our beliefs and institutions, valves and social relationships. These culture changes lead social relationships. These culture changes lead social change.

5. Cultural practices influencing health.

Ans. Health belief and practices are part of every culture. Most ancient and some modern people believe that disease is due to wrath of some supernatural power. Even today, it is believed that venereal disease and leprosy are punishments from god.

Scientific medicine conflicts with folk medicine and their subcultures. Scientific health workers often fail because they do not realize that they must be sympathetically understood. Physicians and nurses must know the subculture with which they are dealing if they are to change the attitude of the patients toward hospital services.

The following cultural practices adversely affect family planning programs:

- Early marriage of the girl extents the reproductive period of the girl child affecting her physical and mental maturity and health.
- Preference for a male child prevents contraceptive practice for spacing, which is needed for regaining the health of the mother and provide her with free time for the first child.
- Low status of woman deprives her of basic nutritional food, shelter, clothing, education, freedom of speech, selection of mate and other important decision-making.
- Taboos in discussing sexual problems openly results in increase in STDs and sex-related health problems.

Following are cultural belief-related to health:

- Getting up early in the morning and taking bath.
- Drinking tulsi water everyday for health.
- Placing jasmine over the breast of postnatal women will suppress the secretion of milk.
- Circumcision of muslim male child prevents urinary tract infection.

- Eating papaya during first trimester and last trimester will induce abortion and premature delivery.
- Purdah system by muslim women causes vitamin D deficiency.
- Giving iron object during convulsion period will reduce intensity of fits.
- Male child is preferred by Hindu parents for performing the last rites.
- Periodic fasting will clean-up gastrointestinal tract. Weekly fasting by Hindu, during the month of Ramzan by Muslim and during lent by Christians.
- Brahman and Vaishya will not consume garlic, onion and non-vegetarian food.
- Avoiding cold food during common cold.
- Drumsticks will not be consumed by some sects.
- Beet root production increases blood production in the body.
- Pregnant women eat mud/ash/chalk powder/lime powder as it enhances the normal development of fetus.

6. Per capita income.

Ans. Per capita income refers to the average income per head in a country. It is obtained by dividing the national income by the total population. As population increases the national income also increases substantially but the per capita income may not increase. It may even fall if the growth of population is too high. It is because the national income gets distributed among the large population. Per capita income of India is very low, as India has low national income but the second largest population in the world. The national per capita income in 1991–92 was ₹ 5583. The 11th five year plan aims at doubling the per capita income.

7. Health functions of the family.

Ans. An addition to the above, a basic family function is to protect the health of the family members and to provide supportive nurturing care during period of illness. In an earlier era, when hospitals were rare, bedridden patients were treated at their homes. It is within the family that members of the family develop their concept of health habits. The family as a social unit, develops a system of values, beliefs, and attitudes about health and illness behavior of its members. Family also transmits health-related cultural traits to next generations.

The health-related functions and task of family are:
  - Provision of adequate, food, shelter, clothing
  - Maintenance of health supporting physical environment at home
  - Maintenance of health supporting psychological environment
  - Provision of resources for maintenance of personal hygiene
  - Health education
  - Promotion of health by nutrition and exercise
  - Health and illness decision-making
  - First aid
- Seeking healthcare, illness care and dental care
- Provision for meeting spiritual needs
- Rehabilitation care
- Interaction and community health personnel.

8. Future of caste system in India.

Ans. Though the influence of caste system is steadily decreasing, it is still very powerful as there is very little change in the attitude and mentality of people. There have been anti-brahmanical movements in Maharashtra, Tamil Nadu, Karnataka and many other states.

There has been a tendency toward formation of caste association particularly among lower caste groups. The elections in India are contested very much on the basis of castes, political parties sponsor only candidates whose caste is the numerous in that area.

The voters in that area are asked to vote for their caste candidates and thus casteism is maintained by the elected leaders after elections are over. Casteism still persists in government services and in legislatures.

9. Family budgeting: For a family income and expenditure.

Ans. Principles of planning a budget

Budget for a month or year depends on:
- Total amount of income
- Different source of the income
- Size of the family
- Status of family
- Provision for the future.

Steps in preparing a budget:
- Record income from all the sources
- List all fixed expenditure and estimated anticipated expenses
- Study the present spending habits of the family and the area, if anywhere the expenditure can be curtailed

- Study the unusual anticipated expenditure to determine whether the satisfaction reached would justify the expenditure
- Find out the best mode of investing at least 15% of the family income on long-term deposits for rainy days.

Advantages of making family budget:

- Budgeting helps the family to spend the money carefully and keeps the expenditure within its means.
- Budget is a good guide for family expenditure.
- It brings balance in current and future expense of the family.
- It prevents family from economic problem.
- Members of family learn value of cooperation.
- It safes the family future and helps in leading healthy and happy life.

10. Some important definitions.

Ans.
- **Culture:** Culture is defined as the training and refinement of mind, taste and manners.
- **Growth:** Growth refers to an increase in physical size of the whole body or any of its parts.
- **Development:** Development refers to a progression in skill and capacity to function.
- **Family:** Family is group of people united by ties of marriage, have blood relation, live together under one roof and use a common kitchen.
- **Family life education:** Family life education refers to those educational concepts and experiences that influence attitudes toward family living; personal relationships and sexual development.
- **Social group:** Social group is a group of people who share some common interest and reason for being together.
- **Social control:** If defined as any influence which the society exerts upon its members for the purpose of providing security to the group as a whole.
- **Social stratification:** It is the process by which groups are ranked in a more or less enduring hierarchy of status.
- **Social security:** Social security has been defined as that security that society provides through appropriate organization against certain risks to which its members are exposed.
- **Health economics:** The word "economics means" housekeeping, it deals with the human relationship in production distribution, consumption and ownership of resources, goods and services.

Behavioral Sciences (Psychology and Sociology) November 2016

Time: 3 Hours **Maximum Marks: 75**

Note: *Attempt any three questions in Section A and attempt all questions in Section B.*

SECTION A

1. **(a) Define perception and write the factors affecting perception.**
   (b) What are the errors in perception?
   (c) Explain the characteristics of mentally healthy person.
   (5 + 5 + 5 + = 15)

2. **(a) Define conflicts and explain the different types of conflict.**
   (b) What are the components of attitude?
   (c) Write the importance of positive attitude for a nurse.
   (5 + 5 + 5 = 15)

3 **(a) Define emotions, enlist the types of emotions.**
   (b) Explain the causes of maladjustment and measures to overcome maladjustment.
   (c) Describe the importance of psychology in nursing.
   (5 + 5 + 5 = 15)

4. **Write short note on following:**
   (a) Drug addiction
   (b) Alcoholism
   (c) Problem solving
   (d) Attitude **(5 + 5 + 5 = 15)**

SECTION B

5. **(a) Explain nature of sociology.**
   (b) Describe importance of sociology.
   (c) Write the important functions of family.
   (5 + 5 + 5 = 15)

6. **Write short notes on any three of the following:**
   (a) Social agencies
   (b) Population explosion
   (c) Culture
   (d) Juvenile delinquency
   (e) Dowry system **(5 + 5 + 5 = 15)**

SOLVED QUESTION PAPER NOVEMBER 2016

SECTION A

1. **(a) Define perception and write the factors affecting perception.**
   (b) What are the errors in perception?
   (c) Explain the characteristics of mentally healthy person.

PERCEPTION AND FACTORS AFFECTING PERCEPTION

Refer paper 2010 question no 3

ERRORS IN PERCEPTION

Refer paper 2010 question no 3

CHARACTERISTICS OF MENTALLY HEALTHY PERSON

- A well-adjusted person has some awareness of his motives, desires, ambition and feelings
- He has a high degree of self-esteem and confidence
- As he is mentally healthy, he will express his emotions in a desirable and controlled manner
- He has capacity to socially adjust
- His intellectual powers are well-developed
- He lives in reality not in a fantasy
- He is always punctual for his duties and does not suffer from forgetfulness
- He is self-confident and optimistic
- He has an adequate sex adjustment and does not suffer from sex abnormalities
- He is well-adjusted and happy with his profession
- He leads a balanced life of work, rest and recreation
- He has the courage for facing failures in his life.

2. **(a) Define conflicts and explain the different types of conflict.**
   (b) What are the components of attitude?
   (c) Write the importance of positive attitude for a nurse.

CONFLICTS AND ITS TYPES

Refer paper 2008 question no 6(c)

COMPONENTS OF ATTITUDE

An attitude has three components:

1. *Cognitive:* What a person knows of it and his belief about it how he perceives events and how he think about them.
2. *Affective:* How he feel about it.
3. *Conative or behavioral:* Behavioral tendency both verbal and non-verbal towards the objects how he acts.

It should be useful to know that a person feels and thinks if one could predict from this, how he is lately to act.

IMPORTANCE OF ATTITUDE FOR A NURSE

Refer paper 2010 question no 4(d)

3 (a) Define emotion and enlist the types of emotions.
(b) Explain the causes of maladjustment and measures to overcome maladjustment.
(c) Describe the importance of psychology in nursing.

EMOTION AND ITS TYPES

Refer paper 2010 question no 2

CAUSES OF MALADJUSTMENT

Refer paper 2007 question no 2

Measures to Overcome Maladjustment

Use defense mechanism for maladjustment, for this refer paper 2007 Q no 3.

IMPORTANCE OF PSYCHOLOGY NURSING

Refer paper 2007 question no 1 (Sec A)

4. Write short note on following:
(a) Drug addiction
(b) Alcoholism
(c) Problem solving
(d) Attitude

DRUG ADDICTION

Refer paper 2007 question no 9

ALCOHOLISM

Alcohol dependence was earlier called as alcoholism.

- **Causes:**
  - Poverty
  - Illiteracy
  - Peer pressure
  - Frustration
  - Ignorance
  - Broken home
  - Family problem
- **Medical complication:**
  - Fatty liver, cirrhosis of liver, hepatitis
  - Gastritis
  - Peptic ulcer
  - Malabsorption
- **Central nervous system:**
  - Peripheral neuropathy
  - Alcoholic hallucinosis
  - Suicide
  - Head injury and fractures
  - Delusion
  - Alcoholic dementia
  - Alcoholic jealousy
- **Social complication:**
  - Accidents
  - Divorce
  - Criminality
  - Marital disharmony
  - Increased incidence of drug dependence
  - Financial difficulties

Treatment

- **Behavior therapy:** The most commonly used behavior therapy is aversion therapy. Many other methods are relaxation techniques, assertiveness training, self-control skills, positive reinforcements.
- **Psychotherapy:** Supportive psychotherapy and individual psychotherapy have been used. The patient should be educated about the risks of continuing alcohol use, asked to resume personal responsibility for change and given a choice of options for change.

Group Therapy

Of particular importance is a voluntary self-help group—AA (Alcholics Anonymous with branches all over the world and a membership in hundreds of thousands.

Deterrent Agents

It is also called alcohol sensitizing drugs, e.g. Disulfiram.

PROBLEM SOLVING

Refer paper 2012 question no 4(c)

ATTITUDE

Refer paper 2009 question no 1

SECTION B

5. (a) Explain nature of sociology.
(b) Describe importance of sociology.
(c) Write the important functions of family.

NATURE OF SOCIOLOGY

Refer paper 2009 question no 6

IMPORTANCE OF SOCIOLOGY

Refer paper 2008 question no 1 (Section B)

IMPORTANT FUNCTIONS OF FAMILY

Refer important theory question no 7

6. Write short notes on any three of the following:
(a) Social agencies
(b) Population explosion
(c) Culture
(d) Juvenile delinquency
(e) Dowry system

SOCIAL AGENCIES

Refer paper 2010 question no 3(a)

POPULATION EXPLOSION

Refer paper December 2008 question no 3

CULTURE

Refer paper 2009 question no 8

JUVENILE DELINQUENCY

Refer paper 2014 question no 3(e)

DOWRY SYSTEM

Refer paper 2014 question no 3(b)

Behavioral Sciences (Psychology and Sociology) October 2015

Time: 3 Hours | **Maximum Marks: 75**

PSYCHOLOGY

Note: *Attempt all questions. Please attempt all parts of the question in sequence.*

1. **(a) Define emotion and enlist different types of emotions.** **5+10 = 15**
   (b) Explain the effects of emotional reactions on health.
2. **(a) Define attitude.** **2+8 = 10**
   (b) Describe the phenomenon of development of attitude.
3. **Write short notes on any three of the following:** **5×3 = 15**
   (a) Perception
   (b) Memory
   (c) Adjustment
   (d) Conflicts

SOCIOLOGY

1. **Write about nursing care of the following:** **2+5+8 = 15**
   (a) Define Group.
   (b) Define Structure and Cycle of group.
   (c) What are the different types of group.
2. **Write short notes on any four of the following:** **5×4 = 20**
   (a) Drug addiction
   (b) Social Problems
   (c) Population
   (d) Family
   (e) Culture

SOLVED QUESTION PAPER 2015

PSYCHOLOGY

1. **(a) Define emotion and enlist different types of emotions.**
   (b) Explain the effects of emotional reactions on health.

Ans. *Refer paper 2010 question no 2*

2. (a) Define attitude.

(b) Describe the phenomenon of development of attitude.

Ans. *Refer paper 2009 question no 1*

3. Write short notes on any three of the following:

(a) Perception (b) Memory

(c) Adjustment (d) Conflicts

PERCEPTION

Refer paper 2010 question no 3

MEMORY

Refer paper 2010 question no 4(c)

ADJUSTMENT

Refer paper 2010 question 1

CONFLICTS

Refer paper 2008 question no 6(c)

SOCIOLOGY

1. Write about nursing care of the following:

(a) Define Group.

(b) Define Structure and Cycle of group.

(c) What are the different types of group.

Ans. *Refer paper 2010 question no 2*

2. Write short notes on any four of the following:

(a) Drug addiction (b) Social Problems

(c) Population (d) Family

(e) Culture

DRUG ADDICTION

Refer paper 2008 question no 73

SOCIAL PROBLEMS

Social problems are the conditions threatening the well-being of society. In a community there are both individual and social problems. When individual problems affect a large number of people, they become social problems. Social problems are solved by social and political social problems. Present day social problems are:

- Prostitution
- Alcoholism
- Drug addiction
- Juvenile delinquency
- Dowry system
- Handicapped
- Unmarried mothers
- Child abuse
- Child labor
- Women abuse

POPULATION

Refer paper 2008 question no 3 (Population explosion) Section-B

FAMILY

It is defined as a group of biologically related individuals living together and eating from a common kitchen.

Characteristics of Family

- **A mating relationship:** A family comes into existence when a man and a women establish mating relation between them.
- **A form of marriage:** Mating relationship is established through the institution of marriage.
- **A system of nomenclature:** Every family is known by a name and has its own system of reckoning descent.
- **A common economic provision:** Every family needs an economic provision to satisfy the economic needs.
- **A common habitation:** A family requires a home for its living.
- **A descent:** All members are connected by common descent.

Types

1. Joint Family
2. Nuclear Family
3. Extended Family

1. **Joint Family:** It is made up of a number of nuclear families which are all related to each other. All of them live in a common house all the men are related by blood. The property is held in common. The senior member controls the internal and external affairs of the family.
2. **Nuclear Family:** The nuclear family is universal in all human societies. It consists of married couple and their children. They have individual freedom. The husband plays a dominant role in the family.
3. **Extended Family:** An extended family may be viewed as a merger of several nuclear families. It occurs when young couples continue to live with their parents and have their own children.

CULTURE

Refer paper 2009 question no 8

Behavioral Sciences (Psychology and Sociology) September 2015

Time: 3 Hours **Maximum Marks: 75**

PSYCHOLOGY

Note: *Attempt four questions including question fifth which is compulsory.*

1. **Define psychology, explain its scope and importance in nursing.** 10
2. **Explain the meaning of personality. What factors affect the development of personality?** 10
3. **Define thinking. What are the different types of thinking?** 10
4. **Describe nature and laws of learning and discuss factors to promote learning.** 10
5. **Write short notes on any three of the following:** 5×3 = 15
   a. Attitude
   b. Frustration
   c. Emotions
   d. IQ Test

SOCIOLOGY

Note: *Attempt any two questions.*

1. **Describe common social problems of society. What measures can be taken to prevent them?** 15
2. **What are the rights and responsibilities of individual in democratic society?** 15
3. **Write short notes on any two:** 7½+7½ = 15
   a. Juvenile delinquency
   b. Population explosion
   c. Functions and needs of family

SOLVED QUESTION PAPER SEPTEMBER 2015

PSYCHOLOGY

1. Define psychology, explain its scope and importance in nursing.

Ans. *Refer question paper 2007 ans no 1 for definition and importance.*
Refer paper Dec 2008 Q No 1 for scope of psychology.

2. Explain the meaning of personality. What factors affect the development of personality?

Ans. *Refer paper Dec 2008 Q No. 5.*

3. Define thinking. What are the different types of thinking?

Ans. *Refer paper 2009 Q No. 2.*

4. Describe nature and laws of learning and discuss factors to promote learning.

Ans. *Refer paper 2008 Q No 4 for definition and factors to promote learning.*
Refer Important Theory Q No. 8 for laws of learning.

5. Write short notes on any three of the following:

a. Attitude
b. Frustration
c. Emotions
d. IQ Test

ATTITUDE

Refer paper 2009 Q No 1 for Definition and describe the development of attitude.

FRUSTRATION

Definition

Frustration is such a condition, in which it is difficult or impossible to satisfy the motivated behavior of person.

Causes

Internal Factors

- **Competition:** Failure in competitions gives birth to frustration.
- **High level of aspirations:** Setting the targets, which are higher than the ability, intellect, capacity of person, increase his chances of failure, which in turn become the cause of frustration.

- **Inborn disabilities:** Blindness, deafness, physical deformities may generate inferiority in the person. Inferiority and failure give birth to frustration.
- **Lack of efforts:** Lack of efforts makes a person incapable of satisfying the goals, as a result, he feels frustrated.

External Factors

- **Natural environment:** It includes earthquakes, heavy rains, less rains, epidemics, etc.
- **Accidents:** Different types of accidents make a person financially, physically, emotionally weak and he becomes prone to failure in life.
- **Political causes:** Censoring the freedom of speech frustrates the person.
- **Social and cultural obstacles:** Various type of rules, norms, traditions, faiths, etc. obstruct the fulfillment of one's desires by putting direct or indirect restrains on the person. As a result, it may give birth to frustrations.

Sources of Frustration

- Environmental forces
- Personal inadequacy
- Conflict between motives.

EMOTIONS

Refer paper 2010 Q No 2.

IQ TEST

Refer paper 2007 Q No 6 (c)

SOCIOLOGY

1. Describe common social problems of society. What measures can be taken to prevent them?

COMMON SOCIAL PROBLEMS OF SOCIETY AND MEASURES TAKEN TO PREVENT THEM

Social problems may be defined as those conditions dangerous to social welfare, about which the members of the society are conscious and feel that they should try to implement some creative program for eradication. This is also true that not only most of these problems are interrelated.

- **Crime:** Delinquency
- **Problems related to unsuccessful social system:**
  - Unemployment
  - Temporary dwelling structures
  - Beggary
  - Broken social harmony
  - Poverty.
- **Illiteracy**
- **Problems of youth:**
  - Unemployment
  - Degradation of moral values.
  - Student unrest and lack of directions
- **Problems of women:**
  - Child marriage
  - Dowry
  - Problems of widows
  - Rape and sexual harassment
  - Prostitution
  - Wife beating
  - Forceful lifting/kidnapping
  - Unmarried mothers.
- **Problem of special groups:**
  - Problems of child
  - Problems of scheduled castes
  - Problems of other backward classes
  - Problems of minority
  - Problems of caste-based reservation
  - Social tradition
  - Desire to marry from recto families.

Measures Taken

- **Health education:** Health education is most important to control these all above social problems. Educate the women about their rights and rights of children.
- **Act:** Various act like child marriage act, MTP act, act against women abuse, dowry system may implement properly.
- **Arrangement of employment:** For this give knowledge and skill to the youth about vocational trainings.
- **Legal actions:** Laws which helps to protect the women abuse, child abuse, delinquency, crime, beggary may implement properly.

- **Health care services:** Be aware the people about various health programs, health agencies which work for the welfare of people without any discrimination of class and cast.
- **Population control:** Education to people about control of population because these all social problems arise from big population size.

2. What are the rights and responsibilities of individual in democratic society?

RIGHTS AND RESPONSIBILITIES OF INDIVIDUAL IN DEMOCRATIC SOCIETY

In the original draft of the constitution there is no clear description of the fundamental duties:

- Follow the constitution, respect its deals, institutions, national flag and national anthem.
- Remember the high ideal which motivated the freedom struggle and follow it.
- Protect the sovereignty, unity and integrity of India.
- Protect the nation and serve it, when called upon.
- Establish equality and fraternity among all citizens rise above all discrimination on the basis of religion, language, area or color, leave all customs, which are against honoring women.
- Understand the proud traditions of our culture and protect it.
- Protect the natural environment comprising of forest, lake, river and wild animals.
- Along with scientific attitude, humanism and attainment of knowledge, add the sentiment of reformation.
- Protect public property and avoid violence.
- Try to go towards progress, in all personal and social activities, so that the nation will go forward and may attain great height.

These fundamental duties/responsibilities are included in constitution just to give knowledge to citizens regarding their civic responsibilities.

Rights

- **Right to equality:** Right to equality is an important basis of democracy in order to provide right to equality to all citizens of India.
  - Discrimination on the basis of religion, caste, sex, etc. is abolished.
  - All can make use of shops, places of recreation, place of worship, wells and rivers.

  - Special provision may be made in favor of women, children, socially and educationally backward classes of citizens.
- **Rights to freedom:** All citizens of India have the rights:
  - To freedom of speech and expression
  - To form association or unions
  - To move freely throughout the country
  - To acquire, hold and dispose of property
  - To assemble peacefully
  - To practice any profession
- **Rights to liberty:** Liberty is the second important pillar of democracy.
  - Freedom of expression
  - Freedom to assemble together peacefully
  - Liberty to form groups and organizations
  - Liberty to travel and stay anywhere in India
  - Protection of life and body.
- **Rights to freedom of religion:** Under this right, religious freedom of every individual is recognized. Individual is free to accept, follow and propagate any religion.
- **Cultural and educational rights:** Every citizen and the interests of minorities are protected. These minorities can own and manage education institutions also.
- **Rights to property**: All to this rights, every individual is free to keep property. State cannot confiscate the property. Under certain conditions, this right is limited. This right has been changed as only legal right.

3. Write short notes on any two:

a. Juvenile delinquency
b. Population explosion
c. Functions and needs of family

JUVENILE DELINQUENCY

Definition

Juvenile delinquency involves wrong doing by a child or young person who is under an age specified by the law of the place concerned.

Causes

- **Physical causes:**
  - Hereditary
  - Age and sex

- Physical defect
- Serious disease
- Excessive physical strength.

- **Mental causes:**
  - Weak mentality
  - Idiots
  - Mental tensions
  - Emotional instability
  - Inferiority or fear
  - Wrong imitations and suggestion
- **Family causes:**
  - Very strict control
  - Over protection
  - Impact of sibling
  - Family without morals
  - Dowry.
- **Other causes:**
  - Illiteracy
  - Industrialization
  - Political criminalization
  - Cultural pollution
  - Obscene films
  - Terrorism
  - Person's environment
  - Population explosion.

Control and Prevention

1. Search for ex-delinquents and reform them.
2. Giving proper guidance and criminals.
3. Setting up special committees to find out criminal circumstance.
4. Provide proper housing and recreational facilities.
5. Improve school environment.
6. Determine punishment according to circumstance of crime.
7. Have separate prisons for different categories of criminals.
8. Have separate prisons for women.
9. Try to make creative change in public opinion regarding crime.
10. Make proper provision for punishment, jail, parole and probation.
11. Take help of sociologists and psychiatrists in crime control programs.
12. Nursing personnel should be taught crime psychology.

POPULATION EXPLOSION

Refer paper 2008 Q no 3.

FUNCTIONS AND NEEDS OF FAMILY

Functions

Refer Important theory Q no 7.

Needs of Family

Refer paper 2008 Q no 2.

Behavioral Sciences (Psychology and Sociology) December 2013

Time: 3 Hours **Maximum Marks: 75**

PSYCHOLOGY

Note: *Attempt any three questions of the following.*

1. **Explain learning. Explain the methods of learning.** 15
2. **(a) What do you understand by personality?** 3+6+6 = 15
   (b) Write the types of personality.
   (c) Explain the factors affecting the development of personality.
3. **(a) Define intelligency.** 2+13 = 15
   (b) What are the different types of intelligency tests?
4. **Write short notes on the following:** 5×3 = 15
   (a) Conflicts
   (b) Problem solving
   (c) Attitude.

SOCIOLOGY

Note: *Attempt any two questions of the following.*

1. **Describe the scope of the sociology and write about its importance in nursing.** 15
2. **Explain the common social problems of the society. How these problems can be prevented?** 8+7 = 15
3. **Write short notes on the following:** 5×3 = 15
   (a) Family
   (b) Population explosion
   (c) Drug addiction

SOLVED QUESTION PAPER DECEMBER 2013

PSYCHOLOGY

1. Explain learning. Explain the methods of learning.

Ans. *Refer paper 2008 question no 4 and important theory question no 8*

2. (a) What do you understand by personality?

(b) Write the types of personality.

(c) Explain the factors affecting the development of personality.

PERSONALITY

Refer paper 2008 question no 5

CLASSIFICATION OR TYPES OF PERSONALITY

Various writers have given classification but according to Dr Jung People classified into two main groups namely extroverts and introverts.

Extroverts

Extroverts are people who take more interest in others and like to move with people. They are friendly and sociable and not easily upset by difficulties. They take decisions quickly and act on them without delay. They are realistic and face the problems of life objectively.

Introverts

Introverts are those who are interested in themselves, their own feelings, emotions and reactions. They are busy in their own thoughts and are self-centered. They are reserved in nature and like to work alone. They are very sensitive and are unable to adjust easily to social situations. Poets, scientists and artists belong to this group.

FACTORS AFFECTING THE DEVELOPMENT OF PERSONALITY

Refer paper 2008 question no 5

3. (a) Define intelligence.

(b) What are the different types of intelligence tests?

INTELLIGENCE

Refer paper 2007 question no 5

DIFFERENT TYPES OF INTELLIGENCE TESTS

Refer paper 2007 question no 5

4. Write short notes on the following:

(a) Conflicts

(b) Problem-solving

(c) Attitude.

CONFLICTS

Refer paper 2008 question no 6 (c)

PROBLEM-SOLVING

Problem-solving is an important kind of thinking. Problem-solving behavior occurs in difficult situation in which a solution is not obtained by the habitual method and past experience in similar situation.

Scientific method of problem solving involve seven steps:

1. **Recognizing the problem:** It is quite possible to have a problem and not be aware of it especially in its early stages.
2. **Defining the problem:** To state exactly what this problem is, that is identifying the problem in definite terms.
3. **Collecting relevant information:** Data from all possible sources that have bearing on the problem. Appropriate tools are gathered, books and magazines collected.
4. **Formulation of hypothesis or possible solutions:** One tries to think of the various possibilities for the solution of one's own problem in the light of the information and his own experiences. Intelligence and other cognitive abilities also help in the formulation of an appropriate hypothesis.
5. **Evaluation of hypothesis or possible solution:** We put into practice the course of action we have chosen as the most appropriate and verify its rightness by the results. All alternative solutions should be closely analysed and evaluated.
6. **Verification:** The validity of the derived conclusion is tested by employing them in solution of various similar problems, if they are found suitable in solving these problems, they are accepted for the current situation also.
7. **Choosing another action if unsuccessful:** If another action is necessary you will have to return to your list of possible solutions and choose again.

ATTITUDE

Refer paper 2009 question no 1

SOCIOLOGY

1. Describe the scope of the sociology and write about its importance in nursing.

Ans. *Refer paper 2007 question no 7 and paper 2009 question no 6*

2. Explain the common social problems of the society. How these problems can be prevented?

SOCIAL PROBLEMS

Social problems are the conditions threatening the well-being of society. Some of the present day social problems are:

- Prostitution
- Drug addiction
- Alcoholism
- Juvenile delinquency
- Dowry system
- Handicapped
- Unmarried mothers
- Child abuse
- Child labor
- Women abuse.

Prevention of Social Problems

For prevention of different types of social problems, the department of social welfare created in 1964. A central social welfare board was set up in 1953. The board is an autonomous body welfare board, consisting of women social workers representatives of the state government have also been constituted and are functioning in all the states. The major program on schemes are as under:

- **Social legislation:** The new constitution of India adopted in 1950, accorded complete equality of rights to women and men. All women now enjoy political rights equal with men. They have the right to vote and get elected at proper age. The hindu marriage act and divorce act have removed the several disabilities women suffered from.
- **Child marriage act:** The child marriage restraint amendment act has raised the age of marriage for girls from 15 to 18 years and for boy from

18 to 21 years. Various other acts have been formulated for the welfare of women, children, workers disabled such as dowry amendment act 1984, maternity benefit act 1961, ESI act 1948, etc.

- **Education program:** Lack of education has been a great hindrance to women's progress, therefore special efforts are taken to raise the literacy rate among women and promote girls education. It is good preventive measure for women abuse.
- **Employment and income generating program:** The government is giving greater attention to the training of women in vocational courses. A new scheme known as STEP to render support to women's employment in various sectors such as agriculture, dairying, animal husbandry, khadi, handloom, handicrafts where women are engaged in work.
- **Hostels for working women:** One of the main difficulties faced by working women is lack of suitable accommodation in a healthy and wholesome environment, keeping in view these difficulties a central scheme of assistance for construction of hostel buildings for working women was started in 1972.
- **Appointment of commission and committees:** The Government of India in order to study the problem of women and for their welfare has been appointing various committees and commission from time to time.
- **Child welfare:** Various schemes and services introduce to solve the problems related to children such as ICDS, aim of this program is to provide various services to the children, e.g. nutrition, immunization, non-formal preschool education, etc.
- **Welfare of the disabled:** The ministry of welfare is implementing program for the early detection, treatment, education and rehabilitation of disabled persons.
- **Welfare of the drug addicts:** Drug abuse is a major social problem in India involving the children and the youth of the country. Any approach to control the problem of drug addiction has to be multi-dimensional involving identification, referal services, treatment, public awareness education, rehabilitation and controlling the supply of illicit drugs.

  The government has promulgated act called narcotic drug and psychotropic substance act which came into force in 1985 to combat this problem.

  Preventive measures include education to target group and the general public through TV, radio, posters, plays, film shows, etc. to create awareness of the problem.

Prevention of Prostitution

The government of India passed an act in 1956 know as 'The suppression of immoral traffic act in women and girls which baned prostitution in its commercialized form. In 1986, the act was amended and referred as 'Immoral traffic act'. It covers all persons, whether male of female, who are exploited sexually for commercial purposes.

3. Write short notes on the following:

(a) Family
(b) Population explosion
(c) Drug addiction

FAMILY

Family is defined as a 'group of biologically related individual living together and eating from a common kitchen'.

Characteristics of Family

- A mating relationship
- A form of marriage
- A system of nomenclature
- A common economic provision
- A common habitation
- A descent.

Types

1. On the basis of structure
   - Joint family
   - Nuclear family
   - Extended family
2. On the basis of marriage
   - Monogamous family
   - Polygamous family
   - Polyandrous family
3. On the basis of authority
   - Patriarchal family
   - Matriarchal family

Family Cycle

- Stage of formation
- Stage of growth
- Stage of retraction
- Stage of disintegration

Family as a Basic Unit for Health Services

Family takes care of health of each family member. The health services to the family are rendered through hospitals, health centers, CHC, etc.

Family pays attention to the health of special groups that is pregnant ladies, lactating mothers, children, aged and handicapped.

POPULATION EXPLOSION

Refer paper 2008 question no 3

DRUG ADDICTION

Refer paper 2008 question no 4 (a)

Behavioral Sciences (Psychology and Sociology) January 2013

Time: 3 Hours **Maximum Marks: 75**

Note: *Attempt all questions. Attempt all parts of questions in continuity.*

SECTION–A (PSYCHOLOGY)

1. (a) Define learning

(b) What are the factors that affect the learning?

(c) Explain the types of thinking. 2+7+6=15

2. (a) What do you understand by the intelligence?

(b) Write down the different types of tests for measurement of intelligence.

(c) Describe the development of intelligent behavior. 2+7+6=15

3. Write short notes on any three of the following:

(a) Problem-solving (b) Intelligence

(c) Learning (d) Attitude 3×5=15

SECTION–B (SOCIOLOGY)

Note: *Attempt any two questions.*

1. (a) Explain society.

(b) Enlist different social problems.

(c) Explain the variations in rural and urban societies. 2+5+5=15

2. (a) Explain the basic needs of the family.

(b) Write about the measures of controlling population. 7+8=15

3. Write short note on any three of the followings:

(a) Parenthood

(b) Social security

(c) Delinquency

(d) Alcoholism 3×5=15

SOLVED QUESTION PAPER 2013

SECTION–A (PSYCHOLOGY)

1. (a) Define learning

(b) What are the factors that affect the learning?

(c) Explain the types of thinking.

DEFINE LEARNING AND FACTORS AFFECTING LEARNING

Refer Paper Dec.-2008 Q. No. 4.

TYPES OF THINKING

Refer Paper Nov. 2009 Q. No. 2.

2. (a) What do you understand by intelligence?

(b) Write down the different types of tests for measurement of intelligence.

(c) Describe the development of intelligent behavior.

INTELLIGENCE AND ITS TYPES

Refer Paper 2007 Q. No. 5.

DEVELOPMENT OF INTELLIGENT BEHAVIOR

Prenatal Diet

During the development period of fetus if the diet of the mother is food, means the development of fetus is also good. Growth and development play a vital role in development of intelligent behavior.

Prenatal Infection

If mother is suffering from an infection during pregnancy, it affects the growth of fetus which leads to many fetal abnormalities which can hinder the development of intelligent behavior.

Socioeconomic Status of Family

If the family is poor, it may lead to poor nutrition and poor hygiene of the family members which can hinder the development of child.

Play

Play also helps the development of muscle, mind relaxation and social interaction.

Prenatal Care and Affection

Parental care and affection play a vital role in the development of a child. If parent's love their child, the child's development may be good but over protection and neglegence may lead to poor development.

Type of School

Schooling also plays an important role in development of an intelligent behavior.

Educational Level of Parents

If parents are educated, their children are also intelligent.

Nutrition

Nutrition also plays a vital role in the growth and development of child. Malnutrition leads to poor development.

Physical and Social Surroundings of Home, etc.

Physical and social surrounding of the child also affect the life of a child. The child from broken family is always mentally disturbed which affects the intelligence level of the child.

3. Write short notes on any three of the following:

(a) Problem-solving (b) Intelligence

(c) Learning (d) Attitude

PROBLEM-SOLVING

Refer Paper January 2012, Q. No. 4(c).

INTELLIGENCE

Refer Important Theory Q. No. 6.

LEARNING

Refer Paper 2008, Q. No. 4.

ATTITUDE

It can be defined as mental predisposition of a person to react in a particular manner to others.

Attitude consists of three components:

- Cognitive
- Affective
- Behavioral

Development of Attitude

Refer Paper 2008, Q. No. 6(a).

Attitude of Nursing

Refer Paper 2010, Q. No. 4(d).

SECTION–B (SOCIOLOGY)

1. Attempt any two questions:

(a) Explain society.

(b) Enlist different social problems.

(c) Explain the variations in rural and urban societies.

SOCIETY

A society may be defined as a group of people who have lived together long enough to become organized and are considered as unit more or less distinct from other human units.

ENLIST SOCIAL PROBLEMS

- Prostitution
- Drug addiction
- Alcholism
- Juvenile delinquency
- Handicapped
- Dowry system
- Unmarried mothers
- Child abuse
- Child labour
- Women abuse
- Poverty.

VARIATIONS BETWEEN RURAL AND URBAN SOCIETY

Rural Community	Urban Community
1. In rural community, the traditional mores are more dominant	In urban society, the traditional mores are less dominant
2. Family control is more	Family control is less
3. There is strong 'we feeling'	There is no we feeling
4. Their relations are personal	Their relations are impersonal
5. Life is simple & uniform	Life is complex & practical
6. The standard of living is low	The standard of living is high
7. Stability is the typical trait	Mobility is the typical trait
8. Family life is more disciplined	Family life is less disciplined
9. There is always community support	There is no community support
10. Family conflicts are less common	Family conflicts are more common
11. There is no overcrowding	There is over-crowding
12. The basis of social life is caste rather than class	The basis of social life is class rather than caste

2. (a) Explain the basic needs of the family.

(b) Write about the measures of controlling population.

BASIC NEEDS OF THE FAMILY

Refer Paper 2008, Q. No. 2.

MEASURES TO CONTROL POPULATION

Control of population is a matter of urgency, not only for socio-economic development but also to prevent low standard of living. The aim of our population policy was to reduce the net reproduction rate of 1 percent.

Family planning or family welfare is the obvious solution to this problem. Family planning refers to practices that help individuals and couples to attain certain objectives.

- To avoid unwanted birth and to bring about wanted births
- To regulate the intervals between pregnancies
- To control the time at which births occur in relation to the ages of parent.
- To determine the numbers of children in the family.

The concept of welfare is basically related to quality of life. As such, it includes education, nutrition, health, employment, women welfare and rights, shelter, safe drinking water.

(a) **Health education:** Health education about spacing methods, benefits of small family size to the eligible couples.

(b) **Easy availability of spacing methods:** To ensure proper supply of contraceptives at the reach of people.

3. Write short note on any three of the following:

(a) Parenthood

(b) Social security

(c) Delinquency

(d) Alcoholism

PARENTHOOD

Planned parenthood or family planning may be defined as children by choice, not by chance. A planned family is a happy family. The government of India is advocating small family norm, that is every married couple should not have more than 2 children.

Advantages

- To raise the standard of living of the country population.
- To avoid unwanted pregnancies and births
- To reduce maternal and infant mortality rates
- To raise the economic standard of the family
- To raise the educational standard of the family
- To raise the health status of country's population
- It helps to have adequate employment opportunities
- It helps in overall development of the nation.

SOCIAL SECURITY

Refer Paper 2008, Q. No. 4(b).

DELINQUENCY

A delinquent is one who shows deviation from normal behavior. He is one who has comitted an offence, e.g. theft, sexual offence, murder, burglary, etc.

- Social maladjustment
- Poverty
- Disturbed home conditions
- Alcoholism
- Drug addiction
- Modern ways of living.

Prevention and Control

The programs for the prevention & control centre around the implementation of the children Act, 1960 & 1986 which provide a specialized approach toward the care, protection, maintenance training & rehabilitation of delinquent children.

ALCOHOLISM

It is a wide social & medical problem. When alcohol is consumed in moderate quantity, it does not constitute a social problem. When an individual takes to drink in excess, he becomes a problem to the family and society. The population groups at great risk are those undergoing rapid socio-economic and cultural changes. Drinking by adult serves as a role model for the young.

Prevention of Alcoholism

Pattern varies considerably the prevention of alcoholism is not easy. The preventive measures include:

- Identification of risk factors
- A widespread public education and discussion
- Investigation of public attitudes
- Strict enforcement of law.

Behavioral Sciences (Psychology and Sociology) January 2012

Time: 3 Hours **Maximum Marks: 75**

Note: *Attempt any three questions from this section. Attempt all parts of question at same place.*

SECTION A (PSYCHOLOGY)

1. **(a) Define psychology.**
   (b) Explain the scope of psychology.
   (c) What is the importance of psychology in nursing? 2+8+5=15
2. **(a) What do you understand by personality?**
   (b) Write the types of personality.
   (c) Write down the factors affecting the development of personality. 3+6+6=15
3. **(a) What is perception?**
   (b) Describe the factors affecting perception.
   (c) What are the errors in perception? 2+8+5=15
4. **Write short notes on any three of the following:**
   (a) Habit formation.
   (b) Adjustment mechanisms.
   (c) Problem-solving.
   (d) Unconscious conflict. 3×5=15

SECTION B (SOCIOLOGY)

Note: *Attempt any two questions from this section. Attempt all parts of question at same place.*

1. **(a) Define sociology.**
   (b) Explain nature of sociology.
   (c) Describe importance of sociology. 2+6+7=15
2. **Write short note on any three of the following:**
   (a) Drug addiction.
   (b) Social agencies

(c) Population explosion
(d) Culture 3×5=15

3. (a) Describe family as a basic unit of health services.
(b) What are the basic needs of family? 8+7=15

SOLVED QUESTION PAPER 2012

SECTION A (PSYCHOLOGY)

1. (a) Define psychology.
(b) Explain the scope of psychology.
(c) What is the importance of psychology in nursing?

PSYCHOLOGY

Refer Paper 2007, Q. No.1.

SCOPE OF PSYCHOLOGY

Refer Paper 2008, Q No. 1.

IMPORTANCE OF PSYCHOLOGY IN NURSING

Refer Paper 2007, Q. No.1.

2. (a) What do you understand by personality?
(b) Write the types of personality.
(c) Write down the factors affecting the development of personality.

PERSONALITY

Refer Paper 2008, Q. No. 5.

TYPES OF PERSONALITY

There are different kinds of personality which are described by different writers, but mainly there are two types of personalities:

1. Extrovert personality
2. Introvert personality.

Extrovert Personality

These people are the excitement seeker and they like variation. They are social in nature and like roaming a lot. Because of such behavioral patterns, they find difficulty in staying within the constant conditions during sideness and feel dull and bore if they have to stay on bed for long time.

Introvert Personality

- Temperament of these type of people is that they remain withdrawn, occupied in themselves, manage stressful situation alone.
- These people avoid excitement and like to stay in constant type of conditions. They dislike variation and to participate in social ceremonies and functions. They think and then react.

According to SHELDON

- **Endomorphic:** They are soft and round people, comfort loving, pleasure seeking, sentimental and socializing people.
- **Mesomorphic:** They have muscular built strong and athletic type, very active, full of energy and less religious. They are aggressive and noisy, achievement oriented people.
- **Ectomorphic:** These people have thin body built, slender and very delicate and fragile. They are sensitive and delicate, intellectual, more religions people. They withdraw.

According to KRETSCHMER

- **Pyknic:** They are fat, round and graceful people, happy, very social, friends, very easily.
- **Athletic:** They have muscular built and strong skeleton, hands and feet large, very active, and aggressive and success oriented.
- **Asthenic:** Thin body built individuals are tall, the skin is dry. A social lacking emotions, dry and unsympathetic look.

FACTORS AFFECTING THE DEVELOPMENT OF PERSONALITY

Refer Paper 2008, Q. No. 5.

3. (a) What is perception?

(b) Describe the factors affecting perception.

(c) What are the errors in perception?

Refer Paper 2010 Q.No. 3.

4. Write short notes on any three of the following:

(a) Habit formation

(b) Adjustment mechanisms

(c) Problem-solving

(d) Unconscious conflict.

HABIT FORMATION

Definition

In simple terms, a habit is a behavior or a set of behavior that you do automatically without thinking and consciously.

Habit Formation Cycle

As it is already said, that habit is a recurrent, often unconcious pattern of behavior which is acquired through frequent repetition. In this way, a habit that starts once, it occurs repeatedly and then a person becomes habitual of it. A habit seems to happen through a cyclical process.

Firstly, it starts with a trigger which can come from our environment or inside ourselves. For example, my boss yells at me. This trigger causes the person to understand its needs. As every human being has needs but the basic human need is to feel understanding of this trigger. But when we deny or repress our needs, we go into the world of thoughts which can be filled with criticisms, judgments, blame and confusion, e.g. anyway, she is so poor decision-maker......................................

I should just quit her office.............................

May be its my fault.......................................

I will never be understood............

Now these thoughts will be surrounded by emotions and hence the emotions arise are often determined by the thoughts that started it. We often avoid our feelings and emotions by suppressing, hiding them or acting them out. When we resist or control our true needs, their thoughts and feelings create pressure inside our system that urgently require relief from this pressure. This relief seeking impulse is often misguided attempt in order to meet the original needs.

But the pressure built-up propels the person to take action in order to alleviate the pressure in our body system and meet the need. It is only short-term pleasure. But in hurry, we often take action not the one that meets our true need. Hence, the person takes alcohol.

Now the person will have judgments about our habits developed, like drinking which is now a new trigger and the cycle begins again. For example, thoughts can be:

I cannot believe, I take too much alcohol.

I am so weak, what a loser I am?

ADJUSTMENT MECHANISM

Defense mechanisms or mental processes are at unconscious level. They are used to reduce anxiety or resolve conflict.

Compensation

It means something given to replace a loss or to make-up for a defect, e.g. a student who fails in his studies may compensate by becoming the college champion in athletics.

Denial

It means to refuse reality, we use denial most often when faced with death, serious illness. Many old people will not easily accept that their mental and physical power are on the decline as they advance in age.

Regression

It means showing childish behavior or behaving in a less mature way, e.g. of backwards. An adult when faced with difficulties of life and wants to protect himself from those difficulties he acts as a child, where he finds less conflicts and less anxiety.

Rationalization

"Making an excuse" In this, we make an excuse by giving a reason different from reality. For example, a student who failed in examination may complain that the hostel atmosphere is not good for study.

Sublimation

It is the channelling of a strong and socially unacceptable drive or urge into a form that is acceptable to society. The most important of these are sexual desire, for example, unmarried women can express repressed sexual desire by becoming a nursery school teacher.

Day Dreaming

Day dreaming is a pleasant thing. It may help us to escape during times of stress. For example, when one is having financial problems, one can escape from them temporarily by planning how to spend an imaginary fortune. Fantasy (day dreaming) may offer temporary relief from pressure. But excessive day dreaming may lead to loss of contact with realities and it may lead to a psychotic disorder called schizophrenia.

Substitution

Substitution is a mechanism which may be employed to reduce tension, resulting from frustration. For example, a student who has not been able to get admission to the MBBS course, may try to substitute it with a course of physiotherapy.

Introjection

In introjection, the values and characteristics of significant person are incorporated in one's personality. For instance, a woman who likes to line in a simple way introjects in her the sophisticated way of living like her husband.

Suppression

It is a device where a conscious effort is made by the individual to dismiss the impulses, feeling and thoughts that are unpleasant to the preconcious mind. For example, a student taking an examination is upset about an argument with her friend but puts it out of her mind so that she can finish the test.

Repression

It is a more complicated mechanism in which unpleasant or unacceptable experiences, emotions and motivation are actively forced into the unconscious and kept there. Unacceptable feelings are unconsciously kept out of awareness. For example, man is jealous of his good friend's success but is unaware of his feelings of jealously.

PROBLEM-SOLVING

It is a process of overcoming difficulties that appear to interfere with the attainment of a goal. It is a procedure of making adjustments in spite of interferences.

Scientific Methods of Problem-solving

- Problem awareness
- Problem understanding
- Collection of relevant information
- Formulation of hypotheses or hunch for possible solution

- Selection of a proper solution
- Verification of the concluded solution or hypothesis.

Factors Affecting Problem-solving

Mainly two factors hinder the development of creative, appropriate and accurate solution.

- Functional fixedness and mental set
- An accurate analysis of problem and evaluation of solution

Some other factors which affect problem-solving are:

- Complexity of the problem
- Lack of resources in the solution of the problem
- Interest
- Motivation and general health status of the problem solver
- Time spent on solving the problem and level of previous training
- Learning of the problem solver.

Nursing Implication of Thinking, Reasoning and Problem-solving

The study of thinking and reasoning would enable the nurse together a wealth of factual material, form the habit of looking for relationships, practice generalizing from facts, look for a central problem, size up the whole situation, avoid prejudices and look for new meanings, avoid hasty generalizations, be tolerant of solutions proposed by others, and cultivate an open mind in all situations. She would also be able to foster correct ways of thinking and finding solutions to problems of her patients, e.g. teaching problem-solving skills to patient recovering from illness.

UNCONSCIOUS CONFLICT

The mental conflict below the level of conscious awareness is called the unconscious conflict. Most of our emotional disorders are caused by our unconscious conflicts. They are often the result of early childhood experiences which have long been forgotten. They follow the process of repression and the formation of complexes.

The conflict even at the conscious level is a painful affair which creates tension in the mind. It should end as soon as possible. It can be ended by following the ID impulses and by ignoring the claims of the ego and the superego or the external world. It can be ended by consciously denying the impulses or urges completely and following the demands of the ego or superego. Another method of ending the conflict is by throwing these impulses into allied channels sanctioned by society and thus obtaining for them a vicarious satisfaction for example, many women who do not marry, satisfy a fundamental wish by becoming midwives or nurses or by directing their own energies to the care and welfare of children. But most people follow neither of these courses. It is difficult to endure the ideas of defeat which result from the denial of our ID desires. Again the ID impulses cannot be satisfied in the face of social opposition. We need suitable potentialities, education, guidance environment. For that normally the conflict is resolved or ended in an average individuals by an actual forcing down of these wishes into the unconscious. This unconscious forgetfulness of the ID impulses or throwing down of these impulses into the unconscious is called repression. These repressed wishes or desires remain active in the unconscious regions of our minds. They slowly gather strength by making alliance with other allied repressed experiences, thus forming an active group. This group of repressed desire working with a common end, i.e. to come back to the level of consciousness is called complex. As soon as complexes are formed, they give rise to a conflict in the unconscious known as the endopsychic conflict.

SECTION B (SOCIOLOGY)

1. (a) Define sociology.
(b) Explain nature of sociology.
(c) Describe importance of sociology.

DEFINE SOCIOLOGY

Refer Paper 2007, Q No. 7.

NATURE OF SOCIOLOGY AND IMPORTANCE OF SOCIOLOGY

Refer Paper 2009, Q. No. 6.

2. Write short note on any three of the following:
(a) Drug addiction
(b) Social agencies
(c) Population explosion
(d) Culture

DRUG ADDICTION

Refer Paper 2008, Q. No. 4 (a).

SOCIAL AGENCIES

Refer Paper 2010, Q. No. 3.

POPULATION EXPLOSION

Refer Paper Dec 2008, Q. No. 3.

CULTURE

Refer Paper 2009, Q. No. 8.

3. (a) Describe family as a basic unit of health services.
(b) What are the basic needs of family?

FAMILY AS A BASIC UNIT OF HEALTH SERVICES

Refer Page 12, Important Theory.

BASIC NEEDS OF FAMILY

Refer Paper 2008, Q. No. 2.

Behavioral Sciences (Psychology and Sociology) November 2010

Time: 3 Hours **Maximum Marks: 75**

Note: *Attempt any three questions from this section.*

PSYCHOLOGY

1. **Define behavior. Discuss motivation and behavioral process of adjustment.** 2+13 = 15
2. **Define emotions. List types of emotions. Explain effect of emotion reactions on health.** 2+4+9 = 15
3. **Define attention and perception. Explain factors affecting attention. Explain errors in perception.** 4+4+7 = 15
4. **Write short notes on any three of the following:** 5+5+5 = 15
   (a) Will and character.
   (b) Individual differences in intelligence.
   (c) Memory and forgetfulness.
   (d) Attitude and nursing.

SOCIOLOGY

Note: *Attempt any two questions from this section.*

1. **Enlist social problems. Describe in detail any two social problems.** 7+8 = 15
2. **Define group. Discuss types, structure and group cycle.** 2+6+7 = 15
3. **Write short notes on any two of the following:** 7 ½ + 7½ =15
   a. Social agencies.
   b. Characteristics of community.
   c. Group behavior and group morale.

SOLVED QUESTION PAPER 2010

PSYCHOLOGY

1. Define behavior. Discuss motivation and behavioral process of adjustment.

BEHAVIOR

The term behavior includes all the motor or contain activities like walking, swimming, dancing, cognitive activities (like thinking, imaging, reasoning, etc.) and effective activities (like feeling, anxious, sad, happy, etc.).

MOTIVATION

Motivation refers to the state within a person or animal that drives behavior toward some goals.

Classification of Motives

Common forms of motives are:

- **Organic physiological/Biological motives:** Hunger, thirst, a desire for sex, temperature regulation, sleep, pain avoidance and need for oxygen.
- **Personal motives:** Need for curiosity, security achievement, the need for self-actualization.
- **Social motives:** Need for power, prestige, recognition, social position and self-assertiveness.
- **Unconscious motives:** These are the outcomes of repressed drives which are tabooed by social customs. But unknowingly, it affects the behavior by means of frustration, short temper and unusual behavior.

Nature of Motivation

It is a process which arouses energy or drive in the individual to proceed in an activity. When the activity is aroused, it fulfils the needs and reduces the drive of tension. This drive of tension is not reduced until the need is fulfilled.

BEHAVIOR PROCESS OF ADJUSTMENT

Adjustment can be possible by changing behavior. Our behavior pattern is developed from four influences –models, roles, feelings, and coping mechanism.

Our past influence is what we learn from the models we see:
They may be our parents, family members, friends, teachers, heroes, community leaders and others we observe. We watch how they act and want to act like them. Second is the role that we held in our family of learning and we learned as a child. Third is the belief attached with each behavior and lastly the influence is coping mechanisms. These are the ways how the person cope or adjust according to the situation, like ego defense mechanisms used.

These behavior changes occur in following four steps:

1. **Listing behavior patterns:** For the successful adjustment, firstly an individual needs to list behavior pattern he want to change.
2. **Listing beliefs relevant to behaviors:** He lists beliefs about the behavior. It means what he thinks or believes for these behaviours. All the beliefs are listed that a person has about the behaviors collect all of them and think about them.
3. **Feelings attached with the particular behavior:** Each beliefs have its own feelings that are relevant to the behaviors. These are pleasure, pain, anger, affection, fear, helplessness.
4. **Pros and cons of behavior:** Finally he looks at the benefits avoiding behavior pattern. He lists all the benefits of eliminating it and the advantages of shifting it.

AIMS of Adjustment

- To maintain active relationship between structural components of society.
- For social reform and social construction.
- To lead a harmonious social life.
- To provide good interpersonal relationship.
- To promote character building.
- To develop social unity.

Methods of Adjustment

An individual should lead a healthy, happy and satisfying life by adopting one or other methods of adjustment.

Direct Method

- Improving efforts
- Compromising methods
- Withdrawal and submissiveness
- Making proper choice and decision.

Indirect Method

By using defense mechanism, the individual will try to adopt himself to the changing situation and accommodating new lifestyles.

Adjustments for Students Nurses

Following are some of the areas where students nurses will need early adjustments:

- Living together in nurses hostel, community life
- Effectively dealing with home sickness
- Healthy personal habits
- Social adjustment
- Accepting responsibility
- Punctuality
- Healthy study habits
- How to take examination
- Evaluation and counseling.

2. Define emotions. List types of emotions. Explain effect of emotion reactions on health.

DEFINE EMOTIONS

The word emotions is derived from latin word 'emovere' means to move away from. Emotion is an acute disturbance of the organism as a whole psychological in origin involving behavior conscious experience and visceral functioning.

Emotions: A mental and physiological state arising through conscious efforts with a wide variety of feeling, thoughts and behaviors.

TYPES

- Primary emotions
- Secondary emotions.

Primary Emotions

These are those emotions that an individual feel first, as a first response to a situation. These are unthinking and instinctive responses that an individual has for example, if we are threatened, we may feel fear. When we hear of a death, we may feel sadness. Typical, primary emotions include fear, anger, sadness, happiness.

Secondary Emotions

These appear after primary emotions, may be caused directly by them, just like primary and secondary colors. They may come from more complex chains of thinking, e.g. news of wartime victory may induce a feeling of joy, but then get tinged with sadness for the loss of life.

EFFECT OF EMOTION ON HEALTH

- **Heart beat:** Emotion reactions result into fluctuations in heart beat. It may rise or fall. These can be measured by ECG.
- **Blood pressure:** Constriction and expansions in blood vessels in emotions can vary the blood pressure contraction, raise the BP whereas expansion leads to lowering of BP.
- **Respiratory rate:** Variation in the rate of breathing develops during emotions. It may rise or fall.
- **Pulse rate:** Emotions also change the pulse rate of a person.
- **Harmonic changes:** Hormonal secretions take place during emotions, level of certain hormones may rise in emotions.
- **Brain waves:** Alertness of brain is observed in the form of waves in day time. Alert stage that requires deep thinking leads to fast waves. As the alertness decreases, the speed of waves also decreases. In emotional reaction such variations in wave speed has been observed. It can be measured by EEG (electroencephalogram).
- **Galvanic skin response:** It refers to bioelectric conductance in skin. Emotions are also accompanied by variations in bioelectric potential in skin which can be measured by biofeedback apparatus for galvanic skin response.
- **Digestive system:** Emotional reaction can result into changes in secretions in digestive tract. That is why some people report digestive troubles during emotions.
- **White blood corpuscles:** These are important components of our immunity system. Any changes in the numbering of these cells can expose

the body for various diseases. During strong emotional reactions, it has been found that the strength of these cells decreases.

3. **Define attention and perception. Explain factors affecting attention. Explain errors in perception.**

DEFINE ATTENTION

Attention is defined as the ability to focus on a person, object or activity for a certain period of time.

Perception

According to Ryburn: It is defined as the process of interpretation of experience of sensation.

FACTORS AFFECTING ATTENTION

Attention is determined by certain factors. These factors are external environmental factors and internal organismic factors.

1. Objective or external factors.
2. Subjective or internal factors.

Objective Factors

- **Nature of stimulus:** Different types of stimuli affect attention in different degrees. Normally light is stronger in affecting the attention. Meaningful stimuli come into attention easily then meaningless stimuli.
- **Size of stimulus:** It has been found that bigger stimuli are attended earlier than smaller stimuli. Take the example of advertising posters pasted on walls where important information is always printed in bigger letters and rest in small because bigger words come into attention quickly.
- **Location of stimulus:** Stimuli closer to sense organs gain attention easily than distant stimuli. For example, students sitting in front seats remain in attention of teacher more than others.
- **Intensity of the stimuli:** Strong stimuli get more attention than weak stimuli. For example, bright light will attract attention more than dim light. Gaudy colors take more attention in comparison to faint colors.
- **Repetition of stimulus:** Repeated presentation of a stimulus takes attention of an individual, e.g. news which is coming repeatedly at news channel will take the attention of people.

- **Sudden change:** Sudden change in stimulus affects attention strongly for example, if a child suddenly stops in a race will take the attention of people.
- **Novelty:** Novel things attract more than usual and common things like new dresses, movies, cassettes, cars take our attention quickly.
- **Movement in the stimulus:** Moving object is more attractive than static stimulus.
- **Rareness:** Those stimuli which are rarely observed, come into attention, quickly, e.g. elephant in city attracts easily.
- **Contrast:** Stimuli that have contrasting characteristics to each other take attention, e.g. very fat and very slim person coming together will gain other's attention.

Subjective Factors

Internal characteristics of a person also affect the attention:

- **Interest:** Stimuli of interest gain the attention of a person easily. For example, new dresses in the market attract girls, new music attracts person having a taste in music.
- **Habit:** Habits also gain attention of people, e.g. a person reads newspaper in the morning will notice the cues related to dropping of newspaper in the morning quickly.
- **Curiosity:** Curiosity about certain things also disposes the attention of person related to those matters easily.
- **Attitude:** Attitudes toward particular groups or persons affect the attention toward those groups strongly. However, weak attitude have weak affect on attention.
- **Practice:** Those tasks or objects on which a person has good practice do affect the attention very weakly, e.g. a star player in cricket may not notice certain news related to cricket.
- **Emotions:** Attention is also affected by emotions, e.g. a frightened person walking alone in night will notice very fine sound too quickly.
- **Temperament:** Attention is also influenced by temperament of a person. A person with religious temperament will be attracted toward religious matters and objects.
- **Needs:** Needs of a person determine the attention. A person hungry for many hours will attract to eatable things quickly.

ERRORS IN PERCEPTION

Illusion

It is wrong perception in the presence of real external sensory stimuli, e.g. snake instead of rope.

- **Illusion caused by stimulus factors:** Horizontal, vertical illusion occur due to the stimulus factor, e.g. to receive your friend at station, you perceive somebody else as your friend from his back.
- **Geometrical illusion:** An observation of the diagram given would lead to every normal person to say that horizontal line 'A' looks smaller than line 'B'.

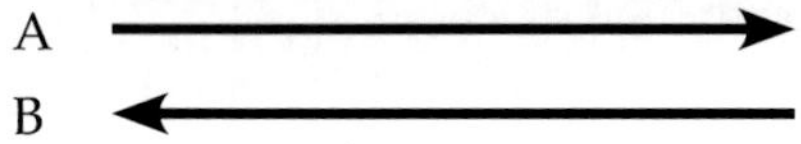

  But actually both the lines are of same length.
- **Fan illusion/Hering illusion:** two horizontal lines are parallel. The distance between 1 and 2 is the same, all the way across the figure. But they appear as unparallel.

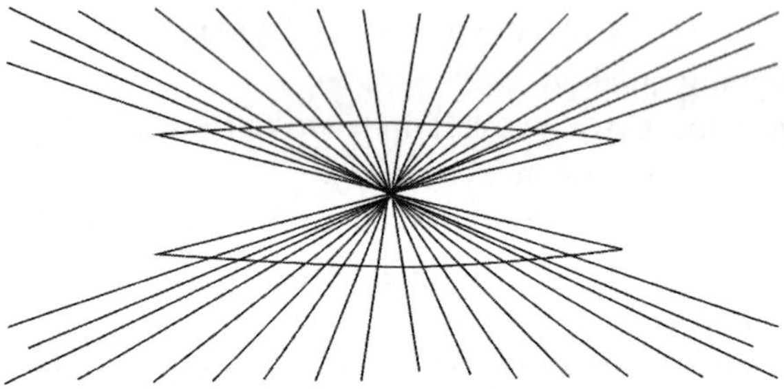

- **Zollner illusion:** All these lines are drawn in a parallel way. But they are not perceived as parallel.
- **Height width illusion:** A tall hat is put in a short vase. The height and width of the hats are equal but one looks taller than the other.
- **Illusion of movement:** When an observer perceives a moving picture when actually the object is not moving.
- **Moon illusion:** The moon looks quite larger near the horizon than when it is over head at its zenith, even though the visual angle subtended by the moon remains constant.

Hallucination

It is a false sensory perception that not associated with real external stimuli. It may be visual, auditory, olfactory, textile, gustatory, but usually visual and auditory are more commonly experienced.

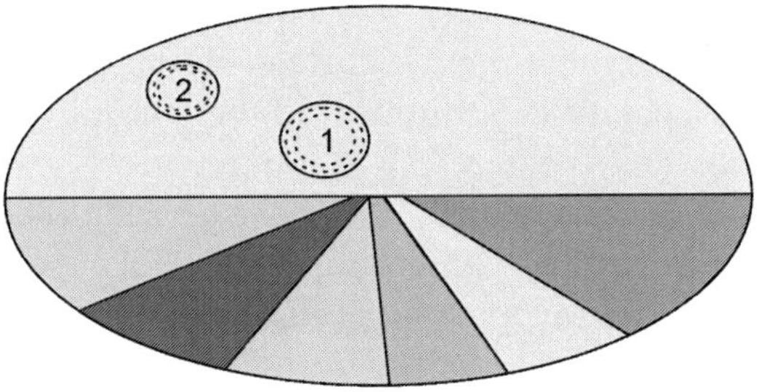

4. Write short notes on any three of the following:
- (a) Will and character.
- (b) Individual differences in intelligence.
- (c) Memory and forgetfulness.
- (d) Attitude and nursing.

WILL AND CHARACTER

Will

Will is the mental capacity of an individual to choose or decide or to do one thing rather than the other. Will is required, when a choice has to be made between two modes of action, two motives, between two or more conflicting behaviors.

Will has three steps namely:
1. Deliberation
2. Vacillation
3. Decision

While engaged in deliberation, the individual who has to decide examines the merits and demerits of the different alternatives available to him. Sometimes the alternatives may be simple and making the choice relatively easy. But on many occasions, the decision-making is difficult and completed on the alternation of equal attraction and strong repulsion.

Then is suspense, hesitation and vacillation and the process is personally painful. After a lot of postponement, a decision in taken at the long last, resolving the conflict between the motives.

Character

Character is one of the acquired factors of human personality, an aspect of our behavior-like habits-skills and attitudes. It is a long-lasting mental structure influencing our conduct and social behavior.

We are not born with character. It is acquired quality. We are born with our physiological and other motives, drives and temperament, gradually we develop skills, habits and attitudes, all these acquired tendencies are called character.

Character and will are related. If we have a strong character, we have abundant will power and no conflicts.

A nurse needs to develop a character which is both psychologically strong and morally good.

INDIVIDUAL DIFFERENCES IN INTELLIGENCE

"Individual difference" is one of the most important characteristics of intelligence.

"Sir Francis Galton 1883" was the first scientist to study the individual difference in a systematic way. He found that people are different from one another in their intellectual ability. The fact behind individual differences is that the two individuals differ in their genetic make-up and also in the environment in which they are brought up.

Even twins also have no similar mental intelligence. There is not only difference in intelligence in different individuals but intelligence varies in the same individual from time to time and situation to situation.

Intelligence and Sex Difference

Various studies have been conducted to find out whether there is any difference in the intelligence levels of males and females in most cases, no significant difference has been noticed.

Intelligence and Social or Cultural Differences

There are no differences according to race and culture. The bright and the dull can be found in any race or caste or cultural group and the differences are due to the influence of environment.

MEMORY AND FORGETFULNESS

Define Memory

It can be defined as recalling the material in present learnt in past, e.g. a student learns a question and then reproduces in exams.

Process of memory takes place into four stages:

1. Learning
2. Retention
3. Recall
4. Recognition.

Types of Memory

It is divided into three types:

1. Sensory memory
2. Short-term memory
3. Long-term memory.

Sensory Memory

It is a memory where memory traces are retained at sense organs only for 1 second. Then memory traces fade away and the material is forgotten.

Short-term Memory

It is a memory where material is retained for 30 seconds only and then it is forgotten, if not transferred to long-term memory.

Long-term Memory

It is memory where the material is retained for many minutes, hours, days, months and years, e.g. date of birth-date of marriage, etc.

Forgetting

It is the failure to recall the material learnt in past.

Causes of Forgetting

- Strength of original learning
- Method of learning
- Nature of material

- Learning under abnormal conditions
- Speed of learning.

Methods to Improve Memory

- **Mnemonics:** The mnemonics are short, verbal devices that encode a long series of facts by associating them with familiar information in the recent part, e.g. colors of rainbow are associated with ROYGBIV.
- **Method of loci:** The method of loci says that you visualize a scene and fit the items to be remembered in that scene. The supposing you want to remember for examination classical conditioning. Then start by imaging a dog, experimental room food, well every person is an experimenter.
- **Rhyming:** Like the method of loci, number and letter peg system is to establish main idea in your long-term memory. A well organized set of images to which the to be remembered items can be linked, e.g. a rhyming system can be used for the number 1 through 10, e.g:
  - One is fan
  - Two is a shoe
  - Three is a tree
  - Four is a door
  - Five is a knife
  - Six is a disk
  - Seven is a pen
  - Eight is a light
  - Nine is fine
  - Ten is men and soon.
- **Narrative stories:** You can make a story and in that you can fit the facts. The important thing for good memory is your motivation and ability to organize the material.
- **Chunking:** If you want to remember a long list of digits, e.g. 2006 1506080 you can break the number into chunks. The first four digits could be remember red as your year of any significant thing that happened in that year, next four digits could be taken as someone's birthday and last three digits as someone's weight.

ATTITUDE AND NURSING

Various attitudes of a nurse that will help in successful nursing practice are listed in following:

- **Respect for the rules and regulation of nursing profession:** Each profession has its own rules regulations depending on the kind of work that is done, similarly nurses around the world have a specific role to play and they have to respect their rules and follow them. This will help them to be successful nursing practioners.

- **Attitudes of pride and desire to grow professionally:** Every nurse should have an attitude of pride not for self, but of the profession. This will help them to succeed very quickly.
- **Interest in solving the problem of others:** A nurse should have the interest to help solve the problems of the patients who are present. Each individual may have the capacity to try and help these people solve their problems.
- **Respect for the opinion and judgment of others:** Each nurse should respect the opinion of the other healthcare workers. This will help the work to go on smoothly and patient will benefit from this.

Other attitudes of nurse that will help them in successful nursing practice are:

- Motivation to search for new knowledge toward effective nursing care through various research projects and literature review. This will improve body of knowledge.
- Respect for the dignity and rights of each person, colleagues or client, family and friends. This attitude of a nurse will make her to become a better person.
- Cooperativeness and respect for the members of health team. This attitude of a nurse will help the work to go on and the patient care to improve.
- Acceptance and understanding of others from different racial and religious background.

SOCIOLOGY

1. Enlist social problems. Describe in detail any two social problems.

SOCIAL PROBLEMS

1. Poverty
2. Prostitutions
3. Drug addiction
4. Dowry system
5. Alcoholism

6. Delinquency
7. Handicapped
8. Child abuse
9. Women abuse.

POVERTY

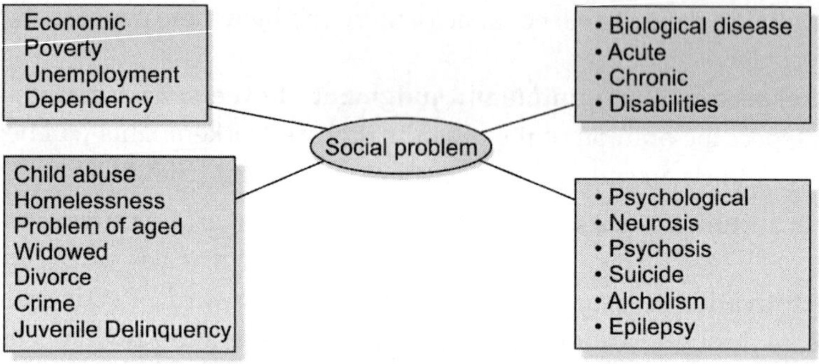

PROSTITUTION

Prostitution in India is a serious social problem. Prostitution is due to:

- Poverty
- Unemployment
- Lack of options
- Stigma and adverse social attitudes
- Family expectations and pressure
- Lack of proper services.

Causes of Prostitution

- Poverty
- Addiction
- Abuse of neglect
- Homelessness
- Family history of prostitution
- Lack of self-esteem
- Peer pressure
- Better life
- Family breakdown
- Loneliness and boredom

- Inability to arrange marriage
- Prior incest of rape
- Psychological causes including desire for physical pleasure
- Lack of recreational facilities.

Laws Related to Prostitution in India

- Suppression of immoral traffic in women and girl act 1956.
- Prevention of immoral traffic act 1956.
- Immoral traffic act 1956.

The immoral trafficking prevention act 1956, the main statue dealing with sex work in India, does not criminalize prostitution or prostitutes per se, but mostly punishes acts by third parties facilitating prostitution like brothel keeping living off earning and producing even where sex work is not coerced.

Institution for Women

Under immoral traffic prevention act 1956:

- **Vigilance/ Protective homes:** There are established act that provide care, treatment, training and rehabilitation to the girls and women. These institutions also admit girls who face the threat of sexual exploitation. The vigilance homes are at Chennai, Madurai, Trichy, Salem, Coimbatore.
- **Rescue shelters:** Rescue shelters established for the purpose of providing custodial care and protection to those who are rescued from commercial sex works shall be admitted in these shelters, providing enquiry before the courts.
- **Unmarried mother's home:** Unmarried girls and women becoming pregnant creates problems for individuals. The result is that such women and girls are subject to ill-treatment. To protect such women and girls, unmarried mother's home have been established.
- **Short stay homes:** A non-government organization provides care and protection to those women and girls who are living in vulnerable situation and are likely to fall victims of abuse.
- **Half-way home:** To provide shelter, education, and vocational training to the girls children who are living in vulnerable situation a half-way home was started under a non-government organization with an accommodation of 25 girls.

DRUG ADDICTION

Drug addiction is prolonged use of drugs. It affects brain functioning and thus on behavior.

Causes

- Inability to cope-up with crisis
- Loss of nearness
- Disappointments
- Feeling of rejection
- Loneliness
- Failures to achieve goal.

Signs/Symptoms

- Headaches
- Tension
- Sleeplessness
- Depression increase.

Prevention

- Parental monitoring and supervision are critical for drug abuse prevention.
- Drug education and information for parents or caregiver about harmful effects of drugs and open opportunity for family discussion about the abuse of legal and illegal substances.
- Focus education for the following programs:
  - Self-control
  - Emotional awareness
  - Communications
  - Social problem-solving
  - Academic support.

2. Define group. Discuss types, structure and group cycle.

DEFINE

By group, we mean any collection of human beings who are brought into social relationship with one another:

- **Primary group:** According to Cooley, it is the nucleus of all social organizations. It is a small group in which a small number of people come into direct contact with one another. They live in the presence and thought of one another. The essential characteristics of primary group are intimate feelings and close identification. Primary groups help in the socialization of the individuals and maintain social control over them. They teach the members to work in the society according to their rules.

- **Secondary group:** Secondary group are those that are relatively a casual and impersonal in their relationship. A secondary group is one which is large in size such as a city, nation, political, labor union, etc. A secondary group is regulated by formal rules. The main purpose is to fulfill a specific function.

Structure of Group

Group structure is developed to regulate the actions of its group members. The group power is the ability to control some aspects of behavior of others by giving them rewards and punishment. Group structure is based on communication system and coordinating the activities of individuals in group. Thus we can classify the structure and its interrelationship through the graphs.

The structure and interrelationship of group (group cycle)

- Two or more persons are the main elements for the formation.

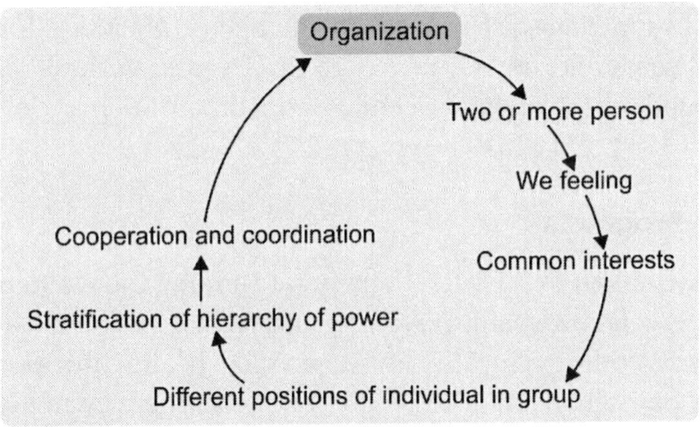

- These persons should have we feeling for the members of group.
- All the group members have common interests or interdependency to fulfill their needs.
- Every individual has his different position or role that he has to play for the welfare of group.
- Stratification of position and hierarchy of power is found in group to perform all higher and lower jobs.

- Cooperation and coordination is found to perform all activities in group members once and start again.

3. **Write short notes on any two of the following:**
   (a) Social agencies.
   (b) Characteristics of community.
   (c) Group behavior and group morale.

SOCIAL AGENCIES

The department of social welfare created in 1964. A central social welfare board was set-up in 1953. The board is an autonomous body welfare board, consisting of women social workers and representatives of the state government have also been constituted and are functioning in all the states. The major programs or schemes are as under:

Social Legislation

- The new constitution of India adopted in 1950, accorded complete equality of rights to women with men. All women now enjoy political rights equal with men. They have the right to vote and be elected at proper age. The Hindu marriage act and divorce act have removed the several disabilities women suffered from.
- The child marriage act has raised the age of marriage for girls from 15 to 18 years and for boys from 18 to 21 years. Various other acts are formulated for the welfare of child and women. Such as dowry amendment act 1984, ESI act 1948, etc.

Education Programs

Special efforts taken to raise the literacy rate among the women's and girl's education. Special programs have been started for women in adult education centers providing education in subjects like health, nutrition, child care and family planning. Including skills like teaching, sewing, embroidery and knitting, etc.

Employment and Income Generating Programs

- The government is giving greater attention to the training of women in vocational courses.
- A new scheme known as STEP to render support to women's employment in various sectors such as agriculture, dairying, animal husbandry,

fisheries, khadi, handloom, handicrafts where women are engaged in work.
- The women development corporations are playing an important role in providing better employment to women so that they become economically independent.

Hostel for Working Women

One of the main difficulties faced by working women is lack of suitable accommodation. Keeping in view, these difficulties a central scheme of assistance for construction of hostel buildings for working women was started in 1972.

Mahila Mandals

The scheme of welfare extension projects was started in 1954 to provide base minimum service to women and children comprising balwadis, maternity, and health services, literacy and social education for women, arts and crafts centers and recreational facilities in rural areas were handed over to voluntary organizations known as mahila mandals in 1961.

Appointment of Commission and Committee

Government has been appointing various committees and commissions from time to time. Such as national committee on the status of women, Indian red cross rotary club and lion's club, family planning association of India, Mahila Mandals, Bharat Sewak Samaj, Indra Gandhi Trust, etc.

Child Welfare

Integrated Child Development Services (ICDS)

This scheme was introduced in 1975. The scheme covers children in the age group of 0 to 6 years, expectant mothers and nursing mothers. AIM of this ICDS is to provide health services such as nutrition, immunization health check-up, education, etc.

Other Programs

Such as crèches, day care centers for children of working women, easily childhood education center, national award for child welfare, celebration of children's day, midday meal scheme for school going children, etc.

Welfare of the old people: There are various organizations and associations concerned with the care and welfare of the aged" help age India, was established in 1978. "Age care India" was established in 1980 with aims and objectives of helping and serving the aged people above 50 years.

Welfare of the disabled: The ministry of welfare is implementing programs for the early detection treatment education, rehabilitation of disabled person.

Welfare of the drug addicts: The government has promulgated an act called narcotic drug and psychotropic substance act which came into force in 1985 to combact this problem.

Preventive measures include education of target group and the general public through TV, radio, leaflets, posters, plays, films, shows, etc. to create awareness of the problems.

CHARACTERISTICS OF COMMUNITY

Each community has some characteristics depending upon the size of community. The following are the characteristics:

- **Permanency:** It means community is that group which lives in a definite geographical area permanently not temporarily.
- **We feeling:** The people in the community have we feeling.
- **Closeness:** The people in community have face to face interaction and free communication. It is more commonly apparent in small communities, small villages and neighborhood.
- **Homogeneity:** The community has similarity in psychosocial characteristics of people living in the defined boundaries of the community. They are similar in language, lifestyle, customs and traditions, etc.
- **Specific name:** Every community has a specific name for its identification in society.
- **Common rules:** Every community has some common rules, every member of community has to obey these rules otherwise there is a provision of punishment. These rules help to control the behavior of its members and to maintain the social system and peace in society.
- **Naturality:** Communities are not made but are natural.
- Wider ends in communities, the people are associated not for the fulfillment of particular end. The ends are wider.

GROUP BEHAVIOR AND GROUP MORALE

Morale is the amount of confidence and enthusiasm which an individual should have as the member of group, every individual in the group possess certain attitudes that are helpful for internal behavior of human group.

Group morale increases the work satisfaction from its total job situation group morale emphasizes on social reaction and concentrates on attitudes toward group values and morales interest, optimistic view, etc. It describes the attitude level in group.

Importance of Group Morale

- To take decision related to group activities.
- To modify or introduce group practice which are conductive to the people in organization.
- To control the difficult situations.
- Through group morale, people can convey their actual feelings, the leader can make special action to ensure the free flow of communication.
- Provides opportunity to the group members to interact with higher authority.
- Create awareness on morale consciousness.
- Man is social animal and he is interdependent on his group members. An individual can fulfill his all needs in groups and feels secure with his mates.
- A group leader can easily make the feeling of morale for its members.

Behavioral Sciences (Psychology and Sociology) November 2009

Time: 3 Hours **Maximum Marks: 75**

Note: *Attempt any* ***three*** *questions from this section.*

PSYCHOLOGY

1. **Define attitude. Describe the development of attitude. (5,10)**
2. **Define thinking. What are the different types of thinking? (5,10)**
3. **What are different factors that affect attention? (15)**
4. **Define personality. What is the importance of will and character in personality? (15)**
5. **Write short notes on: (5x3=15)**
   (a) Approach-avoidance conflict
   (b) Unconscious behavior
   (c) Memory

SOCIOLOGY

Note : *Attempt any two questions from this section.*

6. **Describe the nature of sociology. (15)**
7. **Describe the types, structure and intergroup relationship of group. (15)**
8. **Define community. Give its characteristics and culture. (5, 10)**

SOLVED QUESTION PAPER 2009

PSYCHOLOGY

1. Define attitude: Describe the development of attitude.

DEFINE ATTITUDE

It can be defined as mental predisposition of a person to react in a particular manner to others.

DEVELOPMENT OF ATTITUDES

Formation of attitudes is a development process. It starts developing from the childhood. It can be divided into three stages.

1. Childhood
2. Adolescence
3. Adulthood.

Childhood

Formation of attitude in childhood is based on parent's attitude. Parents approve the children when they express some attitude as parents have, studies also show a very high correlation in the attitudes of parents and children.

For example, parents influence is clearly visible as children always quote their parents as "My papa says or my mama says, etc." on various issues.

Adolescence

It is the most critical period of life and also for the development of attitude of parents. Up to this stage, children have semi liquid attitude so the chance of change in attitude is high during this period of life.

Children have more assess to information from other sources of information at this stage as:

Media, Friends, Education

- Media not only helps in developing new attitude but it can also modify already held attitude acquired from the parents.
- Friends also strongly influence the attitudes of children.
- Education also influences. The education makes attitude of an individual more liberal than an illiterate individual.

As the level of education rises, it results into making attitudes more and more liberal.

Adulthood

In this stage, attitude becomes solid and most difficult to change. This solidification process can be explained with two factors, i.e. commitment and cognitive dissonance. In this age of adulthood, person wants stability in life in different area like in job, in marriage, in religion, etc.

Thus attitude changes from liquid state in childhood to semi-liquid in adolescence and solid in adulthood.

2. Define thinking. What are the different types of thinking?

THINKING

Thinking is a higher mental process which involves verbal, symbols, internal, visual, and auditory images, ideals, concepts and mathematical symbols. Thinking is a cognitive activity.

Types of Thinking

- **Perceptual or concrete thinking:** It is based on perception. Perception is the process of interpretation of sensation according to one's experience. It is also called concrete thinking. It is the simplest form of thinking, small children are mostly benefited by this type of thinking.
- **Conceptual or abstract thinking:** It does not require the perception of actual objects or events. It is abstract thinking and uses abstract ideas. Language plays an important part in conceptual thinking.
- **Creative thinking:** The thinking of scientists or inventors is an example of creative thinking. It is not bound by any established rule. The person himself formulates the problem and he is free to gather evidences and to invent tools for its solution. Creative thinking is aimed at creating something now.
- **Reasoning (Reflective or logical thinking):** Reasoning or problem-solving is one of the best forms of controlled thinking in which the thought process is directed consciously toward the solutions of a problem. Reasoning is the highest form of thinking to find out causes and effects. By this process an individual tries to solve a problem from his past experience. Reasoning may be classified into two types inductive and deductive reasoning.
- **Problem-solving:** It is an important kind of thinking; problem-solving can be done by trail and error or mechanical means. But this method

is time consuming. Problem-solving can also be done through insight, which is a sudden understanding which comes after studying the problems.

3. What are the different factors that affect attention?

Ans. Attention: These factors are external environmental factors and internal organism factors.

OBJECTIVE OR EXTERNAL FACTORS

- **Natural stimulus:** Different type of stimuli light and sound affect attention in different degrees.
- **Size of stimulus:** It has been found that bigger stimuli are attended earlier than smaller, e.g. a poster on a wall with big letters come in attention quickly than small letters.
- **Location of stimulus:** Sense organs gain attention easily to close stimuli than distant stimuli, e.g. students sitting in front seats attention of teacher more than others, that is why some students prefer remain in back seats in classroom.
- **Intensity of the stimuli:** Strong stimuli gets more attention than weak stimuli. For example, bright light will attract more than dull light. Strong sound attracts more than low intensity sounds.
- **Repetition of stimulus:** Repeated presentation of a stimulus attracts an individual which is coming repeatedly at news channel.
- **Sudden change:** Sudden change in stimulus affects attention strongly, e.g. from seminar hall if a person suddenly gets up to leave the hall comes into attention of every person in the hall.
- **Novelty:** Novel things attract more than usual and common things. New dresses, movies, cars attract our attention quickly.
- **Movement in the stimulus:** Moving things attend more attention than stable.
- **Particularness:** Those stimuli rarely observed come into attention quickly, e.g. elephant in city attracts and from any car or bus.
- **Contrast:** Like color contrast, very fat very slim person coming together will gain other's attention.

SUBJECTIVE OR INTERNAL FACTORS

- **Interest:** Interest of a person affects attention like interest in new dresses, new movies, in new music attracts attention of persons.
- **Habit:** Habit, e.g. a person reads a newspaper daily in morning will notice the cues related to dropping of newspaper in the morning quickly.

- **Curiosity:** Curiosity about certain things also gains attention.
- **Attitude:** It has been attitude towards particular groups or persons affecting the attention toward those groups strongly.
- **Practice:** Those tasks or objects on which a person has good practice, do affect the attention very quickly.
- **Emotions:** Attention is also affected by emotions, e.g. a frightened person walking alone in night will notice very fine sounds too quickly.
- **Temperament:** Attention is also influenced by temperament of a person. Things related to religion will be noticed too early.
- **Needs:** For example, a person in need of job will see the vacancy related columns in newspaper easily.

4. Define personality. What is the importance of will and character in personality?

DEFINITION

Personality is the total quality of an individual's behavior as it is shown in his habits of thinking in his attitude, interests, his manner of acting, and his personal philosophy of life.

IMPORTANCE OF WILL AND CHARACTER IN PERSONALITY

Will

Will is the mental capacity of an individual that it chooses or decides or to do one thing rather than the other. Will is required when choice has to be made between two modes of action, between two motives, between two or more conflicting behavior.

Will has three steps:

1. Deliberation
2. Vacillation
3. Decision.

Deliberation

While engaged in deliberation, the individual who has to decide examines the merits and demerits of the different alternatives available to him, sometime alternatives may be simple and making the choice easy. But many time, decision-making is difficult.

The decision is not due to will in a willed decision, the whole self consisting of ideals, sentiments and attitudes or character is in action.

Character

- Character is one of the acquired factors of human personality. An aspect of our behavior like habits, skills and attitudes. It is a long lasting mental structure influencing our conduct and social behavior.
- We are not born with character, it is an acquired quality. Character means a judgment of the individual based on certain qualities. A person has good and bad character depending on whether or nor he is honest and dependable.
- Character and will are related. If we have a strong character, we have strong will and no conflicts. There is no vacillation and decision are taken without delay.
- A nurse needs to develop a character which is both psychologically strong and morally good. Besides such professional qualities as integrity, dignity, mental abilities, self-confidence, a successful nurse must acquire many moral qualities like sincerity, honesty, truthfulness and service. This includes the concept of character both psychological strength and moral goodness.

5. Write short notes on:

(a) Approach-avoidance conflict
(b) Unconscious behavior
(c) Memory

APPROACH-AVOIDANCE CONFLICT

It is the most difficult to resolve because in this conflict a person is both attracted and repelled by the same goal object. We speak of ambivalence as the person has positive and negative feeling about the same events.

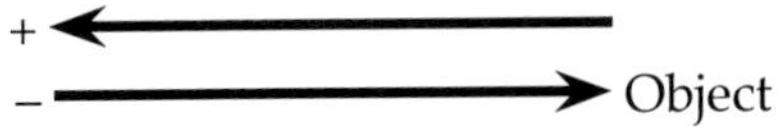

For example, ice cream is delicious but also causes obesity. A man wants to marry a girl for her beauty but some times her educational level is too low. A person picks of the telephone and dials a number, but fearing other person's response, puts the receiver back.

UNCONCIOUS BEHAVIOR

It refers to the influence of repressed thoughts, desires of impulses on our conscious thoughts and behaviors. Freud assumed that free association, dream interpretation and slip of the tongue reveal our unconscious. For example, if ten people witness an accident, we get 10 conflicting reports of the accident. This is because perceptions, prejudices and ideals are unconscious and outside the control of those witnesses.

MEMORY

Simply it can be defined as recalling the material in present learnt in past, for example, a student learns a question and reproduces in exam. Process of memory takes place into four stages:

1. **Learning:** It is the first stage in which material is learnt.
2. **Retention:** Once the material is learnt then it is retained in the form of memory in the mind.
3. **Recall:** Reproduction of learnt material is called recall.
4. **Recognition:** It is the last stage in which the learnt material is presented mixed with new material and the person has to identify the learnt material.

Types of Memory

There are three types of memory:

1. **Sensory memory:** It is memory which is store in sense organs only for 1 second only. And its fade away and forgotten.
2. **Short-term memory (STM):** Where the material is retained for 30 seconds only and then forgotten if not transferred to long-term memory.
3. **Long-term memory:** It is the memory where the material is retained for many minutes, hours, days, months and years.

Levels of Processing

Memory process takes place in three levels:

1. Encoding
2. Storage
3. Retrieval.

- **Encoding:** It is the process of receiving sensory input and transforming it into a code that can be stored.
- **Storage:** It is the process of actually putting the coded information into memory.
- **Retrieval:** It is the process of gaining access to the encoded, stored information, when it is to be used.

SOCIOLOGY

6. Describe the nature of sociology.

NATURE OF SOCIOLOGY

There is a great controversy about the nature of sociology as a science. There are some critics which deny the claim to regard sociology as a science. But these are others who assert that sociology is as much a science as other social sciences. Various characteristics have been mentioned here to explain the nature of sociology.

- Sociology is an independent science.
- Sociology is a social science and not a physical science.
- Sociology is a pure science and not an applied science.
- Sociology is relatively an abstract science and not a concrete science. For example, sociology is not concerned with any particular war or revolution but with wars and revolutions in general as social phenomena, as types of social conflicts.
- Sociology is a general social science and not a special social science.
- Sociology is both a rational and empirical science.
- Sociology, enjoys a preeminent position in the family of social sciences. A knowledge of sociology is considered essential in the field of medicine, nursing, law, business, social relations, administration, social work and other areas of human endeavor.

IMPORTANCE OF SOCIOLOGY IN NURSING

Sociology is important to nursing in the following ways:

- **To understand social life of patient:** It will help the nurse to know social life of the patients. The social environment plays an important part in the causation of health and disease.

  The factors include the cultural values, customs, beliefs, attitudes, religion, education, standard of living, community life, availability of health services, social and political organization.
- **To understand the culture pattern of life:** Sociology will help her to know the deferent culture of each patient. Like in India, have variety of religions, castes, tribes and communities, it is essential to know the culture of each patient. This knowledge is necessary before attempting treatment to make medical and nursing services more effective. For this, knowledge of sociology is essential.

- **To help herself adjustment:** Acknowledge of sociology will help the nurse to adjust herself with the situation in the hospital organization and administration. The nurse must understand how personal goals, values, attitudes and emotional states of doctors and nurses build into life pattern of adjustments and how they influence the doctor nurse relationship in the hospital.
- **To help her maintain good IPR with community:** Nurses working in a community will realize that community is a population made-up of several groups of people living in a certain area. Man is social being and cannot live without the other human beings. Sociology is the study of society and social relations of how people react to one another.

Medical sociology will help the nurse to:
- Recognize the significance of social force in health.
- Understand and appreciate the need to deal with such social process as health values and motivation.
- Organize and administer public health programs as per motivational needs.

7. Describe the types, structures and intergroup relationship of a group.

Ans. According to Cooley, group has been classified into two types.

1. **Primary group:** It is a small group in which a small number of people come into direct contact with one another. The essential characteristics of primary group are intimate feelings and close identification. Primary group helps in the socialization of the individual and maintains social control over them. They teach the members to work in the society according to their rules.
2. **Secondary group:** Secondary groups are those that are relatively casual and impersonal in their relationship. A secondary group is one which is large in size such as a city, nation political, etc. The relations of members are limited in scope his cooperation with his workers is indirect. A secondary group is regulated by formal rules. The main purpose of group is to fulfill a specific function.

GROUP STRUCTURE

In primary group, the group structure is informal unlike in secondary group where the structure is formal and is regulated by formal rules. In the secondary group statues, roles, power and rights of members are clearly defined. In primary group, members are not particular about their rights and powers. The primary group is not well-organized.

But primary group has a well-defined boundary being small in number, the number move within the specified boundary. The secondary group with a large population and has large structure.

INTERGROUP RELATIONSHIP

An individual may belong to many groups without actually meeting any of their other member. In hospital, the nursing staff forms one group of those people who have ever met face to face at any point of time. The nursing staff forms a separate group from the medical staff or the domestic staff.

Who have their own groups. The hospital staff as a whole, however also forms a group with interests and activities concerning all nurses may at same time belong to a professional organization such as TNAI or SNA. These larger groups are the secondary groups. In each group, different demands may be made upon the nurse, sometimes these are conflicting and create anxiety until the difficulties are resolved.

8. Define community. Give its characteristic and culture.

Ans. Community is a human population living within a limited geographical area and carrying on a common interdependent life.

CHARACTERISTICS OF COMMUNITY

- **Locality:** A community is a territorial group. It always occupies some geographic area. Locality is the physical area of a community.
- **Community sentiment:** Community sentiment means a feeling of belonging together and sharing common interests. The members develop a sense of "we feeling".
- **Stability:** A community has not only locality and community sentiment, but has also stability. It is not a temporary group like a crowd or a mob.
- **Size of the community:** There are bigger or wider communities which include small communities like villages, towns, cities or tribes.
- **Regulation of relation:** Every community develop in course of time, a system of traditions, customs, morals and practices, a bundle of rules and regulations to regulate the relations of its members.
- **Dependency:** An individual in a community is physically dependent on community for satisfaction of physical needs.

CULTURE

- Culture refers to the social mechanism of behavior and to the physical and symbolic products of these behaviors.

Accordingly to B Malinowski

It has been defined as the cumulative creation of man. He also regards culture as the hardwork of man and the medium through which he achieves his ends.

CHARACTERISTICS OF CULTURE

- **Culture is social:** Culture is social and not an individual heritage of man. It does not exist in isolation. It is product of society and shared by all the members of the society. No man can acquire culture without association with other human beings.
- **Culture is learnt:** It is not inherited but learnt by man.
- **Culture is shared:** Culture is not something that an individual can possess, e.g. customs traditions, beliefs, ideas, values, morals are shared by people of a group or society.
- **Culture is transmissive:** Culture is transmitted vertically or horizontally and from generation to generation.
- **Culture is continuous and cumulative:** Culture exists as a continuous process. It is linked with the past. Culture is a growing whole which includes in itself the achievements of the past and the present and makes provision for future achievements of mankind.
- **Culture is consistent and integrated:** Culture is an integrated system. At the same time, different parts of culture are interconnected. For example, the value system of society is closely connected with its other aspects like, mortality, religion, customs, traditions and beliefs.
- **Culture is dynamic and adaptive:** Though culture is relatively stable, it is not altogether static. Culture is also responsive to changing conditions of the physical world. It is adaptive.
- **Culture is gratifying:** Culture provides proper opportunities and presents means for satisfaction of our needs and desires. The needs may be biological or social. Through culture, human beings satisfy their needs.
- **Culture varies from society to society:** Every society have its own culture elements, e.g. customs, traditions, morals, ideas, values, belief, practices and institutions are different in each society. It also varies from time to time.
- **Culture is super organic and ideational:** Culture is independent of physical or physiological properties and characteristics. The social meaning of a national flag is not just piece of colored cloth. The flag represents the nation.

Behavioral Sciences (Psychology and Sociology) December 2008

Time: 3 Hours **Maximum Marks: 75**

PSYCHOLOGY

Note: *Attempt seven questions in all. Four questions should be attempted from Part-A and three questions from Part-B. Answer should be brief.*

1. **Explain the scope of psychology.** 10
2. **Define emotions. What is the effect of emotions on our health?** 4, 6
3. **Define and describe adjustment mechanism. List the types of adjustment mechanisms.** 7, 3
4. **Define learning. What are the factors that promote learning?** 4, 6
5. **Explain what you understand by the term personality? List the factors affecting development of personality.** 5, 5
6. **Write short note on any two:** 5, 5
   (a) Development of attitudes.
   (b) Characteristics of the adolescent.
   (c) Conflicts.

SOCIOLOGY

Note: *Attempt any three questions including No. 4 which is compulsory.*

1. **Explain the nature and importance of sociology in nursing.** 7, 8
2. **Describe the basic needs of a family. Discuss the family life education which can be imparted to newly wedded couples.** 7, 8
3. **Explain the term 'population explosion' Discuss its effect on the economy.** 7, 8
4. **Write short note on any of the following:** 5
   (a) Drug addiction.
   (b) Social security.
   (c) Natural resources of the country.

SOLVED QUESTION PAPER 2008

PSYCHOLOGY

1. Explain the scope of psychology.

SCOPE OF PSYCHOLOGY

Psychology studies the human behavior and so, its area and scope is a widespread. Such areas of study in psychology are as follows:

- **General psychology:** It is branch of psychology that deals with the study of behavior of a normal individual in normal life conditions. It includes learning, intelligence sensation, perception, memory, etc.
- **Abnormal psychology:** It is the study of behavior of abnormal individual. Abnormal individuals are those who are suffering from mental disorders, like personality disorders, drug addicts criminal, etc. It includes the study of S/S, cause and treatment of abnormalities.
- **Child psychology:** It has great importance in study of psychological state of child and behavior of children. It studies the physical, emotional, cognitive and moral development of children. It also includes characteristic of child behavior as how they think, feed, perceive and react to different situations in life.
- **Developmental psychology:** It is that branch of psychology that deals with the study of human behavior in the different developmental stages of life from birth to death of individuals. In all the stages, various developmental changes like physical, cognitive, emotional and social are studied.
- **Education psychology:** It is the study of the behavior of individual in education settings. It studies the classroom behavior of student and teacher relationship study methods, teaching methods. It helps to find old study problems of students.
- **Industrial psychology:** In this, behavior is studied in industrial settings. It deals with relationship between man and machine, relationship between management and worker, job satisfaction, etc. It deals with the human problem in industries so as to make the good conditions.
- **Clinical psychology:** It studies the mentally sick persons with special reference to symptoms and treatment of their sickness. Different therapeutic techniques with reference to psychological approaches like psychoanalysis, humanistic, etc. are studied.

- **Comparative psychology:** It studies the animal behavior. As behavior of animals and human is compared so it is called comparative psychology. It is also called animal psychology.
- **Experimental psychology:** This branch of psychology deals with those theories, principle and studies which are obtained using experimental method.
- **Social psychology:** Behavior of an individual in social situation and social groups studies. It includes various subject topics like socialization, leadership, public opinion, social control, crowd behaviors, etc.
- **Physiological psychology:** Structure, functions and mechanism of different body organs and system like nervous system are studied with reference to behavior of an individual. It tend to understand the physiological changes and functioning of bodily mechanism underlying different behavior of human.
- **Community psychology:** It has a broad field where social problems and the attempts of people to adapt to their work and community living are studied in the light of the principles of general psychology.
- **Parapsychology:** The field of psychology that investigates all psychological phenomenon that apparently cannot be explained in terms of scientific laws or principles.

There are many other branches of psychology like:

- Political psychology
- Criminal psychology
- Legal psychology, etc.

2. Define emotions. What is the effect of emotions on our health?

ACCORDING TO GATES

Emotions are episodes in which the individual is moved or excited.

ACCORDING TO BORING AND FIELD

They defined it as emotions resemble the effective responses and have special biological significance for the organism.

EFFECTS OF EMOTIONS ON OUR HEALTH

- **Heart beat:** Emotional reaction results into fluctuation in heart beat. It may rise or fall. These can be measured by ECG.

- **Blood pressure:** Constriction and expansion of blood vessels in emotions can vary the blood pressure. Constriction raise the blood pressure whereas expansion leads to lowering of blood pressure. It can be measured by sphygmomanometer.
- **Respiratory rare:** Variation in the rate of breathing develops during emotions. It may rise or fall.
- **Pulse rate:** Emotions also change the pulse rate of a person.
- **Harmonic change:** Hormonal secretion takes place during emotions. Level of certain hormones may rise in emotions.
- **Brain waves:** Alertness of brain is observed in the form of waves. Relaxed wakefulness is accompanied by moderate speed waves and during deep sleep. There are slow waves. As the alertness decreases, the speed of waves also decreases.
- **Digestive system:** Emotional reaction can result into change in secretion of digestive tract. That is why some people report digestive troubles during emotions, e.g. peptic ulcer, asthma.
- **White blood corpuscles:** These are important components of our immunity system. Any changes in the numbering of these cells can expose the body for various diseases. During strong emotional reactions. It has been found that the strength of these cells decreases.

Other Some External Changes

They consist of facial expressions, bodily movements, gesture, voice disturbance and other. Our face gets flushed up in anger and becomes white and pale in fear, eyes drop down in sadness, break in the voice may denote deep sorrow, a loud, sharp and high pitched voice is there usually in anger. Postures and gestures also reveal emotional tension.

A person who is angry makes others angry some time conational harmful, some time beneficial.

3. Define and describe adjustment mechanism. List the types of adjustment mechanism.

DEFINITION

As the body protects against physical danger or distress, similarly the individual has devices for protecting himself against psychological danger and distress.

ADJUSTMENT MECHANISM

These protective devise are known as defense or adjustment mechanism.

- **Adjustment:** It is the process by which an individual maintain a balance between his needs and circumstances that influence the satisfaction of these needs.
- Adjustment mechanism refers to unconscious processes that defend a person against anxiety.
- The human being uses these mechanisms to solve some conflicts.
- Adjustment mechanisms enable a person to resolve the conflict and reduce the stress and anxiety associated with it.
- When more adaptive measures to resolve the conflicts are not available to the individual, their mechanisms help him to live comfortably without having to face very difficult problems.
- All of us use adjustment mechanism at many times in our normal behaviors.
- When used moderately the area is harmless and help us face conflicts and frustration easily and protect our ego. Excessive use of these mechanism is harmful as they do not solve conflicts and frustrations.

LIST OF DEFENSE MECHANISMS

These can be divided into two groups:

1. Successful
2. Unsuccessful.

Successful

- Repression
- Rationalization
- Compensation
- Substitution
- Sublimation
- Intellectualization.

Unsuccessful

- Suppression
- Displacement
- Projection

- Conversion
- Reaction formation
- Denial
- Fantasy
- Regression
- Fixation.

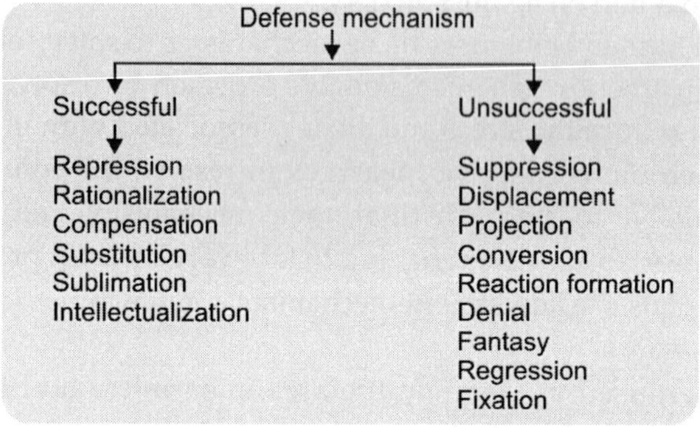

4. Define learning. What are the factors that promote learning?

ACCORDING TO GATES

He defined learning as a modification of behavior through practice and experience.

ACCORDING TO GUILFORD

He defined learning as a change in behavior as a result of experience.

LEARNING IS A SELF-ACTIVE PROCESS

It is a purposeful and goal-directed process that stimulates the interest a person can learn only through his or her reactions to situation.

FACTORS PROMOTING EFFECTING LEARNING

- **Motivation:** The stronger and clearer motive in learning, and interest shown by the learner in learning promote learning. As a result of it, the learning is more permanent.
- **Intelligence:** Intelligence helps the person to understand things to know the relationship between things, to judge correctly. Level of intelligence affects process of learning. The person with more IQ level, learn easily then the mentally retarded.

- **Maturation:** We learn things when we are mature to learn them, e.g. the child should be mature physically before he can learn to walk or run, e.g. a child cannot learn cursive writing unless the has developed the neuromuscular coordination for learning that.
- **Physical condition of the learner:** Physical health of the learner is an important factor-sensory defects, malnutrition, lose of sleep and fatigue are some physical factors that affect learning.
- **Good working conditions:** Factors like lack of fresh air, light, comfortable place, proper temperature and noise affect learning process.
- **Mental health of the learner:** Mental health of the learner is another important factor. Worrier, fear, feeling of loneliness affect learning process. If the learner has no self-confidence, he cannot learn properly, self-respect and praise are very useful in making learning process effective.
- **Length of working period:** The period of work should not be too short or too long. Very short learning period affects the concentration of a person and very long learning period leads to mental fatigue and reduces learning.
- **Learning situation:** Physical facilities for learning as institution, textbooks teachers, audio-visual aids promote learning.
- **Age:** Age factor also affect learning, children learn quickly than older.
- **Physical health:** As physically handicapped person, e.g. deaf and dumb, chronically sick cannot learn.
- **Learning method:** Method or material affect learning. Active learning is better than passive learning. If learner gets involved in learning, is learnt better and speedily.
- **Nature of learning material:** Meaningfulness, length, difficulty level of learning material affect the speed of learning, easy material is learnt speedily than difficult material.
- **Practice:** Practice again and again helps in more learning.

5. Explain what you understand by the term personality? List the factors affecting development of personality.

PERSONALITY

- The word personality is derived from greek word person, the mask used by actors in greek drama.
- Personality is sum total of personal qualities.
- Personality is defined as total quality of an individual's behavior as it is shown in habit of thinking, attitude, interest, manner of acting, etc.

According to Boring

He defined personality as the integration of those systems of habits that represent one individual adjustment to his environment.

FACTORS AFFECTING DEVELOPMENT OF PERSONALITY

- The physiological factors.
- The environmental or social factors.
- The mental or psychological factors.

Physiological Factors

- This is concerned with the physique of the individual like strength, size, looks and constitution. An attractive physical appearance helps to create self-confidence.
- According to physique, larger people have impressive personality and develop a tendency to dominate. A small person may try to compensate for his physical inferiority by being hardworking.

Environmental or Social Factors

- Social aspects of an individual and environment affect personality. The influence of the school and the playground, the social codes and social roles which the individual has to play in the family environment and in the community affect the personality. If the home is characterized by an atmosphere of peace, love, mutual understanding, the child is likely to develop a self-confident and secure personality. If he is overprotected he is going to develop an overdependent personality.
- A good school develops the child educationally and mentally. It provides opportunities for receiving knowledge, thinking and reasoning and developing a broader outlook on life.
- Other social factors that influence our personality are the cinema, the newspaper and the radio.

Mental or Psychological Factors

- They include our motives, acquired interest, our attitudes, our will, our intellectual capacities such as intelligence, reasoning, attention, perception and imagination.
- Intelligence will help him in making adequate adjustments and in collecting facts and understanding relationship. All this will have a beneficial effect on the growth of personality.

6. Write short note on any two:
(a) Development of attitudes
(b) Characteristics of the adolescent
(c) Conflicts.

DEVELOPMENT OF ATTITUDES

Formation of attitudes is a development process. It starts developing from the childhood. These can be divided into three stages.

1. Childhood
2. Adolescence
3. Adulthood

Childhood

Formation of attitude in childhood is based on parent's attitude. Parents approve the children when they express some attitude as parents have, studies also show a very high correlation in the attitudes of parents and children.

For example, parents influence is clearly visible as children always quote their parents as "my papa says or my mama says etc." on various issues.

Adolescence

It is the most critical period of life and also for the development of attitude of parents. Up to this stage, children have semiliquid attitude so the chances, of change in attitude are high during this period of life.

Children have more assess to information from other sources. Other sources of information at this stage are:

Media, Friends, Education

- Media not only helps in developing new attitude but it can also modify already held attitude acquired from the parents.
- Friends also strongly influence the attitudes of children.
- Education also influence. The education makes attitude more liberal than illiterate individual. As the level of education rises, it results, into making attitudes more and more liberal.

Adulthood

In this stage, attitude becomes solid and most difficult to change. This solidification process can be explained with two factors, i.e. commitment and cognitive dissonance. In this age of adulthood, person wants stability in life at different areas of life in job, in marriage, in religion, etc.

Thus attitudes change from liquid state in childhood to semiliquid in adolescence and solid in adulthood.

CHARACTERISTICS OF ADOLESCENT

During this period, physical, social and mental changes develop in adult after childhood.

Physical Changes

In the end of later childhood, sexual changes of puberty begins, socondary characteristics develop, e.g.

- Enlarged hips
- Breast develop in girl
- Muscular development and voice change in boys
- Both sex begin to grow pubic hair.

Social Changes

There is a development of a sense of identity regarding occupational, familiar and social role. This requires a stable, loving home life and wise, mature parents, who understand the needs of their children. This helps adolescents to feel good about themselves and this will promote a good relationship.

CONFLICTS

When two or more motives arise in mind at a same time is called conflict.

Or

It is a condition when two or more goals come into competition with each other in such a way that achievement of one goal is blocked by other goal. It is called conflict.

Types

There are four types:

1. Approach-approach
2. Avoidance-avoidance
3. Approach-avoidance
4. Multiple approach-avoidance conflict.

Approach-approach

It is a condition when two or more equally attractive goals come into competition and only one can be achieved for example, a child after divorce of parents has both relations, important but he has to choose one, in that situations conflict arises.

Mother ←—— Child ←—— Father
+Positive   +Positive

Avoidance-avoidance

It is a type of condition where two or more than two goals appear negative and painful but only one can be avoided. For example, a child has not finished his homework. If he will go to school, teacher will punish him but if he stays at home, he will be punished by parents. If he avoids one goal, other is also painful and dangerous for him.

Approach-avoidance

It is the most serious type of conflict. It is a condition where a goal has both negative and positive characteristics. Positiveness of goal attracts for achievement but the negativeness repels. For example, an individual has got a good job which he wants to join but does not want to go away from home. But both conditions cannot be separated.

Multiple Approach-avoidance Conflict

- Sometimes the goal may have many attractive and adversive characteristics then it is called multiple approach-avoidance conflict.
- For example, a girl wanted to marry a boy, who is handsome, intelligent, and rich but after marriage. She will have to sacrifice her career and parents.

SOCIOLOGY

1. Explain the nature and importance of sociology in nursing.

NATURE OF SOCIOLOGY

There is a great controversy about the nature of sociology as a science. There are some critics which deny the claim to regard sociology as a science, but these are others who assert that sociology is as much a science as other social sciences. Various characteristics have been mentioned here to explain the nature of sociology:

- Sociology is an independent science
- Sociology is a social science and not a physical science
- Sociology is a pure science and not an applied science
- Sociology is relatively an abstract science and not a concrete science. For example, sociology is not concerned with any particular war or revolution but with wars and revolutions in general are social phenomena, are types of social conflicts
- Sociology is a general social science and not a special social science
- Sociology is both a rational and empirical science.

Sociology, enjoys a preeminent position in the family of social sciences. A knowledge of sociology is considered essential in the field of medicine, nursing, law, business, social relations, administration, social work and other areas of human endeavor.

IMPORTANCE OF SOCIOLOGY IN NURSING

Sociology is important to nursing in the following ways:

To Understand Social life of Patient

- It will help the nurse to know social life of the patients. The social environment plays an important part in the causation of health and disease.
- The factors include the cultural values, customs, beliefs, attitudes, religion education, standard of living, community life, availability of health services, social and political organization.

To Understand the Culture Pattern of Life

Sociology will help her to know the different cultures of each patient. Like in India, there is a variety of religions, castes, tribes and communities. It is essential to know the culture of each patient. This knowledge is necessary before attempting treatment to make medical and nursing services more effective. For this, knowledge of sociology is essential.

To Help herself-adjustment

A knowledge of sociology will help the nurse to adjust herself with the situation in the hospital, organization and administration. The nurse must understand how personal goals, values, attitudes and emotional states of factors and nurses build into life pattern of adjustments and how they influence the doctor nurse relationship in the hospital.

To Help her to Maintain Good IPR with Community

Nurses working in a community will realize that community is a population made-up of several groups of people living in a certain area. Man is a social being and cannot live without the other human beings. Sociology is study of society and social relations as how people react to one another. Medical sociology will help the nurse to:

- Recognize the significance of social force in health
- Understand and appreciate the need to deal with such social processes as health values and motivation
- Organize and administer public health programs as per motivational needs.

2. Describe the basic needs of a family. Discuss the family life education which can be imparted to newly wedded couples.

BASIC NEEDS OF FAMILY

- **Physical needs:**
  - Food
  - Shelter
  - Clothing
  - Safe physical environment.
- **Biological needs:**
  - Freedom from communicable diseases
  - Control of insects and vectors
  - Planned parenthood
  - Control of rodents.
- **Psychosocial needs:**
  - A happy home
  - Safe-working environment
  - Freedom from poverty
  - Adequate medical care
  - Care of special groups
  - Social security.

FAMILY LIFE EDUCATION TO NEWLY WEDDED COUPLE

Family life education which is given to a new wedded couple should be in the form of awareness about their importance in the society, of sexuality, marriage and planned parenthood, so that this knowledge will contribute to the individual's ability to cope both with social stage and with relationships in the society as a citizen, spouse and parent.

Objectives

- To avoid unwanted births
- To bring about wanted births
- To regulate the intervals between pregnancies.

Married life is not easy also it is not one of the most stressful relationship between a man and a woman but the best available.

Motivation to Couple for Parenthood

- To motivate the woman to conceive
- Pressure of traditions by parents
- To encourage the mother regarding motherhood
- To motivate the couple to sincerely wish to become parents.

Preparation for Parenthood

- The basic goal of parenthood is to promote the mother physically and psychologically.
- To educate the mother how to do care during pregnancy and after delivery.
- To teach the couple about special needs of pregnancy like good nutritional diet.
- Encourage mother to take proper nutritional diet to fulfill the requirement of baby.
- To educate the parents to give more attention toward growth and development of child after his birth.
- To educate the parents to fulfill all requirements of child during pregnancy, infancy and toddler.

Other knowledge about basic needs, growth and development of child.

Attitude toward Pregnancy

First a couple has to take decision that whether they are ready for the child or not. In some cases if wife's attitude has been unfavorable, it improves after the baby birth. If both are ready, it is easy for lady to carry pregnancy. If woman is mentally prepared for pregnancy then she can easily cope with physical changes during pregnancy and enjoy the married life.

Maternal Role

During pregnancy, mother's health plays very important role because child's health is depending on mother's health. Educate the mother about promotion of health and prevention from disease to establish a good relationship between mother and child.

Planning about Children's Education

All parents have a dream to give better education to their children. Now a days, education is very expensive but government is providing many facilities like education loan. In this way, parents can give better parenthood to children and they can fulfill their responsibilities.

Planning for Future

For the better parenthood, parents plan the needs of children according to their age group. Parent's responsibilities are not only upto childhood but up to the child becomes independent. Parents have to save some money for their future also.

Understanding Child's Temperament

The child's temperament affects the parenthood. Parents are able to understand the changes in child's behavior during their period of growth and development.

These all help the newly wedded couple to live happy married life.

3. **Explain the term 'population explosion' Discuss its effect on the economy.**

DEFINITION

When the population rate of the country increases too high in comparison to natural resources of the country and thus disturbing the natural balance is known as population explosion.

Effect of Population Explosion on the Economy

Population growth has adversely affected our per capita income. The growing population not only effects the economical condition of society, but also social religious living and health condition of the society.

Economical Conditions

There are various areas where the economy of a country is disturbed due to population growth. The main effects of population explosion on economy includes:

- The per capita income of general people decreases which directly leads to poverty. The increasing poverty results in improper and inadequate nutrition and poor hygiene conditions of people leading to increased sickness rate. The money power is wasted on treatment of sickness, again leading to more poverty states. Thus it is clear that population explosion adversely affects the economy of a country.
- There are limited vacancies which lead to unhealthy competition to get jobs. Resulting in unemployment problem.
- There is more starvation, crimes and increased rate of corruption.
- There is increase in many social problems like beggary, delinquent behavior, prostitution, disruption of law and other situation, etc.

Health Problems

Due to population explosion, there is an increase in congested areas and slums in atmosphere and environment gets polluted. The factories, chemicals transportation have also increased, due to which the air, water and land get polluted, so ultimately resulting in large number of diseases both mental and physical for example, TB, eye infection, STD, etc. Because of stress and strain people are also mentally affected.

Effect on Living Conditions

There will be housing problem, not enough schools, so literacy rate will also fall. Over crowding in homes, hospital, buses and trains, there will be strain on public utility services such as electricity, water supply and sanitation, living standard of people will fall down. So, many problems will arise due to increase in population rate so, in order to overcome this, it is necessary to check population growth by adapting different methods.

Need for Population Control

If the population rate is not controlled, it will result in disaster. It gives rise to many problems like:

- Unemployment
- Crime
- Lack of facilities, like food.

Water supply, housing, loss of natural resource, soil erosion, ozone layer, depletion, green house gases effect to atmosphere, decreased standard of living.

Thus it is very important to have some control on the fast growing rate of population to make the general people happy and self-sufficient and for overall development of the country.

4. Write short note on any of the following:

(a) Drug addiction.

(b Social security.

(c) Natural resources of the country.

DRUG ADDICTION

Drug addiction is defined as a state of periodic or chronic toxication determinental to individual and society, produced by the repeated intake of habit forming drugs, e.g.

- Opium
- Charas
- Ganja
- Bhang
- LSD
- Cocaine
- Chloroform
- Morphine.

Drug addiction follows the following criteria:

- **Psychological dependence:** There is an over powering desire or compulsion to take the drug and obtain it by any means.
- **Physical dependence:** There is physical or bodily dependence over the drug. When the drug is withdrawn, the patient shows withdrawal symptoms such as irrational and violent behavior, nausea, vomiting, diarrhea, watering of eyes and nose, etc.
- **Development of tolerance:** There is a tendency to increase the dose.

Preventive Measures

- **Education:** Proper education should be given to college students and youth about the danger of drug abuse through mass media.
- **Legislation:** There should be proper implementation of laws by the government, restriction on availability of drugs and alcohol should be there.

- **Solution of social problems:** Solution to social problems should be found out. Social problems like one's employment, broken homes, etc. should be solved, which can become the cause of drug addiction.

Camps

There should be arrangement of camps and seminars for youth regarding ill-effects of drug abuse by the government. Youth should be included in some recreational and creative activities like going to gym, listening to music in order to divert the mind toward same productive activity.

Parents Education

Parents should be educated about observation of their children because under influence of peer, they can undergo the habit of drug addiction.

SOCIAL SECURITY

Social security has been defined as the security that society provides through appropriate organization against certain risk to which its members are exposed. The risks covered in most countries by social security are sickness, invalidity maternity, old age, and death.

Social Security for Industrial Workers

These are:
- The workmen's compensation Act 1923
- Control maternity benefit Act 1961
- Employees state insurance Act 1948
- The family pension scheme 1971.

Social Welfare in India

Social welfare movement has joined ground in India like many other nations of the world. The department of social welfare was created in 1964 and is responsible for general social welfare including nutrition program for children and pregnant mothers.

Welfare Programs

- Programs for the welfare of children
- Composite programs for women and children
- Programs for the maladjusted group

- Programs for the welfare of women
- Programs for the physically handicapped person, e.g. blind, deaf, mentally challenged, etc.
- Program for the welfare of backward classes.

Central Welfare Board

The central social welfare board was set-up in August 1953. It surveys the need and requirements of social welfare organization in the country. It distributes funds to voluntary social service or organization for strengthening, improving and extending the existing activities in the field of social welfare and for developing raw programs.

Women Welfare New

The department of women and child development created in 1985 formulated and implemented the policies and programs relating to women and child welfare.

Government of India Programs

The Government of India has lunched a number of programs to eradicate the poverty and unemployment in India. The main are following:

- Community development program or 2nd October 1951
- Integrated rural development program during the 6th five-year plan
- National rural employment program
- Rural landless employment guarantee program
- Training program for rural youth for self-employment
- Jawahar Rojgar Yojana (April 1989).

Voluntary Organization

Important voluntary organizations are:

- The Indian red cross society
- Bharat sewak samaj
- The kasturba samaj
- The kasturba memorial fund
- Lions club
- Ramakrishna mission
- Indian council for child welfare
- All India women's conference
- The all India blind relief society.

NATURAL RESOURCES OF THE COUNTRY

India is very rich in natural resources and manpower. The main natural resources are:

- **Agriculture:** India's economy is heavily dependent on agriculture. It accounts for nearly 44% of national income and provides employment for nearly 67% of India's population.
- **Forestry:** It is other natural resource of country, nearly 231 of total land area of the country is occupied by forests. It is source of timber, bamboo, resins, rubber, dyes, honey, etc.
- **Fisheries:** India has a vast sea coast. The marine products feed the locals and earn foreign exchange. 18 million fishermen draw their livelihood from fisheries. Out of total production of 28.5 lakh ton, 11-tons come from inland fisheries and 17.5 lakh ton from the sea.
- **Water resources:** Surface water: Total resources of surface water are estimated 168 million, of which 33% is in loss due to evaporation, 22% seeps into the soil and 45% flows in to river for irrigation.

  Underground water of 36 million hectares seeps down the soil, to lakh is absorbed by the upper layer helping the growth of agriculture crops.
- **Power:** Commercial sources of energy consist of coal, natural gas, hydroelectric power and nuclear fuel accounting for 45% of all energy in India. Non-commercial sources of energy like firewood, charcoal, dried cow dung account for 35% of total power consumption.
- **Manpower:** The greatest natural resource of the country is its manpower. The people of India account for about 16% of world's population.

Behavioral Sciences (Psychology and Sociology) October 2007

Time: 3 Hours | **Maximum Marks: 75**

PSYCHOLOGY

1. Give a suitable definition of psychology. Why is it needed for nursing profession?
2. What is adjustment? Give an outline of the various causes of maladjustment.
3. Explain five adjustments of defense mechanisms.

Or

4. What is the difference between illusion and delusion? Explain factors influencing perception.
5. Define intelligence. What are the different type of intelligence tests?
6. Write short notes on two:
   (a) Law of effect.
   (b) Methods of reducing forgetting.
   (c) Intelligence quotient.

SOCIOLOGY

7. Define sociology and describe its scope.
8. Explain with any five examples, operating at social and economic levels which may badly influence human adjustment and well-being.
9. What measures can be undertaken to prevent drug addiction? Explain.

SOLVED QUESTION PAPER 2007

PSYCHOLOGY

1. Definition of psychology and its importance in nursing.

DEFINITION

Psychology is derived from two greek words "psyche and logos" "Psyche" means soul or spirit and "logos" means knowledge or study. It means, it is the study of soul. Psychology is defined as the scientific study of behavior and mental process.

IMPORTANCE IN NURSING PROFESSION

Psychology has become an integral part of every profession including nursing. It is very important for every nurse to understand the psychology because it helps the nurse in following ways. It will help her understand herself.

A nurse herself is a human being. She may have certain strengths and weaknesses in herself, knowledge of psychology helps her to identify these strong and weak points in herself. With the understanding of psychology, she controls own anxiety before dealing with the patient. She will realize how she makes decision in her life and how she solves her problems. This will lead her life to more productivity and relate with others efficiently.

It will Help her Understand herself

A nurse herself is a human being. She may have certain strengths and weaknesses in herself. Knowledge of psychology helps her to identify these strong and weak points in herself with the understanding of psychology, she controls own anxiety before dealing with the patient. She will realize how she makes decision in her life and how she solves her problems. This will lead her life to more productivity and relate with others efficiently.

It will Help her to Understand Patients

A patient might be suffering from some biological as well as psychological problems. Knowledge of psychology helps her to understand these psychological abnormalities of patients and she can handle accordingly. These patients are different from normal patient so psychology helps her to handle them carefully. Every patient cannot be treated in the same way, if a nurse understands the individual differences in patient then it is possible to give them proper care.

It will Help her to Understand Others

Nursing job does not limit the interaction of nurse with patients and doctors only but she also has to deal with the other person who is related with patient, this will lead to personal and professional adjustment. She will understand them better and this way she will achieve greater success in interpersonal relationship.

It will Help her to Understand Close Relationship of Body

- She will recognize how her emotions affect her body and she will recognize the same for her patient.
  An understanding of psychology can be a great help to a nurse to become a good health teacher to explain to the patient and relatives:
  - The nature of diagnostic examination, finding and treatment
  - After care and rehabilitation therapies.
- Psychology has removed a lot of superstitions in the diagnosis and treatment of mental sickness. It also contributes to many therapeutic measures including behavior therapy, play, group and shock therapy, etc.

2. What is adjustment? Give an outline of the various causes of maladjustment.

ADJUSTMENT

Adjustment is defined as the series of methods, techniques or processes by which an individual tries to meet the environmental, spatial or psychological changes and maintains a satisfactory balance with his world. This is also called adaptation.

Personal and Professional Adjustment by Nurses

Professional nursing means the person requires training and higher education to do practice in the profession of nursing. As a person becomes a nurse, she becomes a member of a profession and will have to learn to adjust to the profession as well, it is called professional adjustment.

CAUSES OF MALADJUSTMENT

Maladjustment is a symptom of ill-health. The chief causes of maladjustment include the following:

- ***Frustration:*** When the basic needs of an individual are not satisfied, there is a tendency of frustration. The degree of frustration depends upon the unmeet needs. It is not the solution, it leads to maladjustment behavior of individual.

- *Tension:* Worry and tension upset mental balance. Certain organic diseases of the body such as hypertension, peptic ulcer, etc. are due to worry and tension.
- *Insecurity:* Insecurities like poverty, children's problem belonging to poor homes, etc. Feeling of insecurity leads to unsatisfied basic needs and it leads to maladjustment.
- *Environmental factor:* It can produce maladjustment even in healthy person. Many social causes lead to maladjustment, for example:
  - Broken homes
  - Death of parent
  - Separation of parents
  - Step parents, poverty
  - Alcoholism
  - Severe punishment
  - Lack of discipline
  - Lack of moral teaching
  - Ignorance about child care
  - Too many children and absence of facilities
  - Urbanization, etc.

  The living status of the individual also effects and health may cause maladjustment in some conditions. To control the maladjustment, is necessary to identify the stress factor and promote positive adaptation.

3. Explain five adjustments of defense mechanism.

Ans. As human body develops its own system to protect against physical danger or distress, similarly the individual devices for protecting himself against psychological dangers and distress. These protective devices are known as ego defenses or defense mechanisms or mental mechanisms.

FIVE ADJUSTMENTS MECHANISMS

- **Compensation:** It means something given to replace a loss or to make up for a defect, e.g. a student who failed in studies, may compensate by becoming the college champion in athletics.
- **Denial:** It means to refuse reality, we use denial most often when faced with death, serious illness. Many old people will not easily accept that their mental and physical power are on the decline as they advance in age.

- **Regression:** It means showing childish behavior or to behave in a less mature way for example, of backwards. An adult when faced with difficulties of life and wants to protect himself from those difficulties he acts as a child, where he finds less conflicts and less anxiety.
- **Rationalization:** "Make an excuse". In this, we make an excuse and give a reason different from reality. For example, a student who failed in examination, may complain that the hostel atmosphere is not good for study.
- **Sublimation:** It is the channeling of a strong and socially unacceptable drive or urge into a form that is acceptable to society. The most important of these are sexual desires, for example unmarried women can express repressed sexual desires by becoming a nursery school teacher.
- **Day dreaming:** Day dreaming is a pleasant thing. It may help us to escape during times of stress. For example, when one is having financial problems, one can escape from them temporarily by planning how to spend an imaginary fortune.

  Fantasy (day dreaming) may offer temporary relief from pressure. But excessive day dreaming may lead to loss of contact with realities and may lead to a psychotic disorder called schizophrenia.

4. What is the difference between illusion and delusion? Explain factors influencing perception.

Delusion	Illusion
1. Delusion is defined as a false belief, e.g. a person has a false belief that he is a prime minister (In grandeur type of delusion and he tries to give order as a leader to other)	1. It is wrong or false perception because of wrong interpretation stimuli, for example of a rope in the dark is perceived as a snake. Other example, a moving dry leaf in dark can be perceived as a moving insect
2. Delusion have many types like: • Delusion of persecution • Delusion of reference • Delusion of guilt • Nihilistic delusion • Delusion of grandeur • Delusion of self-accusation	2. There is no type of illusion present

FACTORS INFLUENCING PERCEPTION

- Perception always takes places with the help of sense organs. They may be visual, auditory, olfactory, muscular, factual perception, etc.
- There are many factors which influence perception:

Subjective Factors

Perception is also determined by certain organismic factors which depend upon the internal characteristics of person, determining factors may not be same to all individuals because of subjectivity in it.

- **Motives and needs:** Motives of a person affect the perception of a person, e.g. a hungry person will perceive eatable things more quickly than others. Needs also determine this perception, an unemployed person will perceive vacancy related news easily. A person who is in need of money, will give attention on loan facilities than others.
- **Mental:** Mental readiness can also affect the perception. For example, memorizing of certain questions during examination days gets very fast.
- **Interest:** Perception also influences the person's interest. For example, subject is according to student's interest, they perceive very quickly than uninterested topics.
- **Emotions:** Emotional state also affects the perception. If a person has any emotional disturbance like fear, anger, etc. he perceives the things in wrong way. In anger, the perceptual ability often gets decline.
- **Values:**Values help in the evaluation of many things happening around us. So perception is also greatly affected by it. For example, a child of alcoholic father will perceive alcohol as a normal thing, whereas child belonging to religiously orthodox family perceive it as dangerous and harmful thing.
- **Habits:** Habits can also affect the perception. Habits direct perception in a particular way any place with trees and flowers will be perceived as a garden. A person with white apron will be perceived as a doctor or nurse because it is our habit to see them in this dress.
- **Familiarity:** The things which are familiar are perceived more quickly than others for example, we can recognize our parents, brother and sister from far distance and even in dim light conditions.
- **Attitude:** Attitude toward others can influence perception about them, people with positive attitude toward exercise and diet will perceive news related to health more quickly.
- **Past experience:** Past experience about anything help the person in quick perception in second attempt.

  For example, small children, before going to school, learn some simple words from parents and when same words are taught by teacher in school, they learn easily.

OBJECTIVE FACTORS

External characteristics of stimulus shows affect on perception, these factors are: Size, intensity, color, contrast, novelty, movement, etc.

5. Define intelligence. What are the different type of intelligence test?

DEFINITION

These different definitions have been given by different all:

- **According to Thorn Dike:** Intelligence is the ability to give response that are true.
- **According to Terman:** Intelligence is the ability to carry on abstract thinking.
- **According to Bin:** Intelligence is a goal directed behavior.

DIFFERENT TYPE OF INTELLIGENCE TEST

There are different type of intelligence tests which are classified into four categories by psychologists:

a. **Verbal intelligence test:** In these, test language is used and written questions are framed which can be answered orally or in writing. These test can be administered on educated people only. Illiterate and abnormal people cannot perform on these tests. These tests can be applied individually or on a group, e.g. Binet Simon intelligence test.

b. **Nonverbal intelligence test:** Language is not used in these tests, diagrams, wooden blocks, pictures, etc. are used. These tests can be administered to educated, illiterates, abnormal persons. These tests can be given individually or in group form. Nonverbal tests are conducted by expert psychologist, e.g.:
   - Cattell's culture-fair intelligence test
   - Bhatia's battery of intelligence test.

c. **Individual intelligence test:** These tests can be administered to an individual at a time. These tests are usually utilized in clinical settings. Administration of these tests require skilled and trained persons only. Tests can be verbal or nonverbal.
   For example, Alexander pass along intelligence test.

d. **Group intelligence test:** Such tests can be used for a group at a time. These tests are usually in competitive exams. Administration of these tests do not require trained or skilled person, e.g. army alpha test:

Test can be categorized into 2 more types:

a. **Speed test:** These tests have such type of items which may not vary in difficulty level, these tests are time fixed. An individual has to perform in a limited time. For example, Cattell's culture fair test, Jaloto's group test.

b. **Power tests:** These tests have items which vary in difficulty level. Subject can take enough time but it is instructed to finish as soon as possible, e.g. Alexander's pass along intelligence test.

Intelligence quotient (IQ): In the measurement of intelligence, IQ level has a great importance, IQ gives us such standard score which remains constant irrespective of age and it is easy to understand the level of intelligence of a person.

6. Write short note on two:

(a) Law of effect.
(b) Methods of reducing forgetting.
(c) Intelligence quotient.

LAW OF EFFECT

As per law, if some response is rewarded with some prize or benefit, it will be learnt. For example, if a child is given chocolate for helping others, the child will do that helping behavior again and again. It will be learnt on other side if some behavior is punished, it will be left unlearned. If a child is punished for stealing, the child will stop that bad habit. However, this second part of law has some objections. If punishment does helping control of bad habits then all the criminals after punishment in jail must have left crime. But it does not happen. Later on studies have proved that punishment is effective only for those behavior which are newly learnt. Behavior which is turned into strong habits, is not controlled by punishment.

METHODS OF REDUCING FORGETTING

There are different methods for reducing forgetting including:

Proper Learning Method

Use of proper learning method like training, practice, motivation, demo can improve memory and reduce forgetting. Learner's interest, span of attention and right learning methods have vital roles to play in reducing forgetting.

Memory Tricks

With a systematic and organized set of images or words with which we are very familiar and can provide reminders. It is the technique of memory improvement.

Memory Pegs

Memory pegs help us to reduce forgetting. Memory pegs with the analogy of a clock room in mind, the reminder clues are called memory pegs. To hang to be remembered items example the letters of the word vibgyor can be used and "PEGS" on which to hang the names of rainbow colors.

The Method of Loci

The word loci means "places". The memory pegs of this system are parts of your images of a scene. The scene can be street, for example you want to remember for examination, classical conditioning.

Rhyming System

Think of the words that rhyme with numbers like one is a bun, 2 is shoe, 3 is tree and so on. Now when you have a list to remember, you can associate the items on the list with your images of the numbers.

Make a Story

If you have a list of unrelated items to remember, a useful memory device is to relate the items in a made-up story. The story starts with the first item on the list and each succeeding item is included in that order.

Chunking

By chunking method, you can also reduce forgetting. If you want to remember your credit card number, you can break the numbers into chunks, by this you cannot forget the numbers.

INTELLIGENCE QUOTIENT

Intelligence is the ability to give response that is true. William stern the German psychologist introduced the concept of IQ. IQ is obtained when the mental age is divided by the chronological age, which is the actual age of the person in years and multiplied by 100.

$$IQ = \frac{MA}{CA} \times 100$$

Imagine a 10 years old child scores a mental age of 12, his IQ will be:

$$IQ = \frac{MA}{CA} \times 100 = \frac{12}{10} \times 100 = 120$$

Thus, the bright child has an IQ of 125 while the slower child has an IQ of 83.

Any person will reach a maximum IQ at about 18 years. Depending upon favorable conditions such as higher education and challenging learning experience, the IQ may increase slightly till age thirty. After 30, the IQ does not change except that it decreases slightly with old age. There is no difference between IQ of men and women.

When children grow into adults, the CA will constantly increase but MA will change very little, this is as per the formula,

$$IQ = \frac{MA}{CA} \times 100$$

Then IQ will become lower and lower for a person growing older and older. The result of IQ test for adults are compaired with the test results of other adults of the same age and not with same person's chronological age. This is called the deviation IQ.

SOCIOLOGY

7. Define sociology and describe its scope.

DEFINITION

- "Sociology is the science of society or of social phenomenon."
- "Sociology may be defined as a body of scientific knowledge about human relationship."
- According to King, it is "general science of society. "
- **According to Park and Burgess:** "Sociology is the study of collective behavior."

Scope of Sociology

Since, sociology is so elastic a science, it is difficult to determine where its boundaries begin and end. The scope of sociology being so wide, an effort has been made to divide its study into different fields. The main fields are:

- **Sociological theory:** This includes the study of sociological concepts, principles and generalization.

- **Historical sociology:** This includes the study of past social institutions and origin of present ones.
- **Sociology of family:** It studies the origin, growth, functions, kinds and nature of family.
- **Sociology of community:** It is the study of community.
- **Special sociologies:**

  It Includes the following:
  - Educational sociology
  - Economic sociology
  - Cultural sociology
  - Medical sociology
  - Political sociology
  - Industrial sociology
  - Social sociology
  - Military sociology
  - Sociology of law
  - Sociology of social stratification.

The sociologist studies various characteristics of any society like human habits, customs, maintenance or order and peace and geographical nations, so that he is able to understand man, his social relationship, his behavior patterns group interactions, social order and social structure. It is useful in many ways like in social pathology, the focus is on social problems like prostitution, alcoholism, drug addiction, etc. He also studies the problems of industrial organization.

Medical and paramedical professions seek the help of sociology to see the social factors causing illness. It helps us in gaining knowledge about ourselves and our society. In this way, it can be said that the scope of sociology is very wide.

8. Explain with any five examples, operating at social and economic levels which may badly influence human adjustment and well-being.

Ans. There are many factors which influence the main factors include:

- **Economic status:** Economic status of a person can greatly affect the adjustment and well-being of individual. For example, a person having poor-socioeconomics status would not be able to manage with daily activities, not able to provide good nutritional food to his family members, not able to provide good health services so he and his family can become the victim of many diseases and thus, the process of adjustment can be derailed.

- **Marital status:** Early marriage of girl effects her reproductive health, physical and mental maturity. Preference for male child prevents the use of contraceptive methods and in this way having no spacing between children and it causes bad effect on woman's health.
- **Illiteracy:** The literacy rate also affects human adjustment and well-being because the illiterate people are not aware of any health problems and their causes and routes. So, they easily become patient of various diseases. Illiterate people are not aware about diet and its necessary nutrients which protect health. Lack of knowledge disturbes well-being.
- **Social myths:** Social myths and misconceptions are also the major factors contributing to ill-health of human being, e.g. some people think that tuberculosis, leprosy, and smallpox are due to wrath of supernatural power and past sins. That's why they do not take medicine and these myths become the cause of death for them.
- **Dowry problem:** Dowry is becoming the major problem of India. It is also affecting human adjustment and well-being. It leads to low status of women, suicide is commitment by young girls and parents come under debt and this leads to many dowry deaths.

9. **What measures can be undertaken to prevent drug addiction? Explain.**

DRUG ADDICTION

Addiction is a condition caused by excessive or continued use of habit forming drugs. The drug addiction is a serious problem of our country leading to many socioeconomic problems affecting the normal structure of the society and general well-being of the community person.

Preventive Measures

There are many measures which can be undertaken to prevent drug addiction. The main measures are following:

- **General education:** Education plays very vital role to prevent drug addiction. It includes education to people and students about the bad effects of drug on body. For spreading education, various methods like mass media, role play, films, charts, etc. are used. Education to avoid bad habits will help in eradicating drug addiction.
- **Control of social problem:** Various social problems like unemployment should be solved because unemployment can become the cause of family

stress and family stress can lead to drug addiction. So solution of social problems should be find out.

- **Counseling:** Proper counseling should be done of those who undergo drug addiction because of any stressful situation.
- **Parent's education:** Parents should be educated about keeping keen observation of their children because under the influence peer, children can undergo habit of drug addiction, specially those living out from house in hostels, so proper guidance and education to parents can solve the problem. Parents should teach their children about the side effects of drugs used in excessive.
- **Educational camps:** There should be arrangement of camps and seminars for the youth regarding ill-effects of drug abuse by the government.

  Youth should be included in some creative activities like going to gym, listening to music, etc. in order to divert their mind toward some productive activity.
- **Drug de-addictions camps:** These should be organized by government in civil hospitals and in other community organizations and proper treatment and follow-up should be done by sufferers. They should be encouraged to take care of their health and avoid taking drugs and use their abilities and capabilities for the good of the nation.
- **Legislation:** There should be proper implementation of laws framed to prevent drug addiction by the government. Proper license checking of the chemist shop should be there and only license holder should be allowed to practice and sale the drugs only on doctor's prescription.

  The government had promulgated an act called the narcotic drug and psychotropic substance act which came into force in 1985 to deal with drug addiction. This should be implemented forcefully into the society.